FOOD SOLUTIONS
Eczema

Recipes and Advice to Provide Relief

Patsy Westcott

hamlyn

Safety note

This book should not be considered a replacement for professional medical treament. A doctor should be consulted on all matters relating to health; particularly in respect of any symptoms which may require diagnosis or medical attention. While the advice and information in this book are believed to be accurate, neither the author nor the publisher can accept any legal responsibility for any injury or illness sustained while following the treatments and diet plan.

First published in Great Britain in 2000 by
Hamlyn, a division of Octopus Publishing Group Ltd
2–4 Heron Quays, London E14 4JP

This revised edition published 2005

ISBN 0 600 61054 3

EAN 9780600610540

A CIP catalogue record for this book is available from the British Library

Printed and bound in the United Kingdom by Mackays of Chatham

10 9 8 7 6 5 4 3 2 1

Contents

	Introduction	7
1	The skin	11
2	Understanding eczema	23
3	Controlling the symptoms	45
4	Orthodox medical treatment	65
5	Complementary treatments	77
6	Food and eczema	99
7	Exclusion recipes	121
8	Healthy eating	173
	Glossary	223
	General index	227
	Recipe index	237

Introduction

Many of us think of eczema as a condition affecting only children. In fact, although some types are more common in childhood, the condition can affect anyone at any age – man, woman or child. Although eczema and dermatitis are not life-threatening, they can cause severe misery and disruption to the sufferer's everyday life and that of their family. In severe cases life may revolve around keeping the house allergen-free and in daily skin care routines to alleviate symptoms. Unfortunately, people with eczema often report that their doctors are not always as sympathetic as they could be.

This book is designed to help you understand the causes of this skin condition and to provide ways to help you manage it more effectively rather than letting it rule your life. It explains the different types of eczema and dermatitis so you can pinpoint the specific type affecting yourself or a family member, enabling you to devise a tailor-made treatment plan. This book can also help you discover the potential triggers and irritants that spark off a bout of eczema and provides simple, down-to-earth advice on ways to avoid them or to minimize their effects.

It also outlines the huge number of treatments available for the relief of eczema, from over-the-counter creams and moisturizers to medical treatments which have been devised especially to treat eczema. You'll also find a rundown of some of the complementary therapies that have been found by many people to be helpful in controlling eczema, together with details of how to find a complementary practitioner and what to expect when you pay them a visit.

Eczema is a chronic condition, one that persists for a long period of time, and as with any chronic disease it is important to look at your lifestyle and understand how various aspects of it may affect the condition of your skin. Because diet and nutrition are so important in keeping us fit and well and in building a strong, healthy immune system, you will find advice on how to plan a nutritious diet that will help you to cope with stress – in itself a frequent factor in triggering eczema – and keep your skin healthy.

Diet can also play a part in triggering some kinds of eczema. In this book you will find more specific information on how to identify the food or foods that may spark off your eczema and how to devise a healthy, nutritious diet that avoids the offending foodstuffs as well as providing you with all the essential nutrients. This can be quite a challenge, so, to make it easier for you, chapters seven and eight include a wide range of delicious, nutritious recipes designed both for overall good health and for people who react to certain types of food.

Eczema cannot be cured but it can be managed. By using the appropriate medical treatment and by looking at your lifestyle and diet, and taking what steps you can to look after your skin and keep it healthy, you can take charge of your condition. And that is what this book is all about.

1 The skin

If you or a member of your family has any of the different types of eczema, you are probably only too aware of the skin and the way it reacts to the outside world. This chapter explains what the skin does and how it works as it protects the body from day to day. This will help you understand better what goes wrong with the skin in eczema and why it affects you in the way it does.

Most people without a skin complaint never give their skin a second thought. Yet the stuff that covers our bodies is a truly remarkable and complex material which performs many different functions. It is strong but flexible, waterproof but absorbent, elastic, washable, anti-bacterial, self-repairing – and designed to last a lifetime. So just what is this amazing material and how does it work?

What exactly goes wrong with the skin when affected by eczema? And is there anything you can do to help your skin stay healthy and prevent this condition?

Protect and survive

It is true to say that the skin is the most complex organ in the whole of the human body. It is also the largest, covering an area of around 2 sq m (2⅖ sq yd) and performing a host of important functions that are literally vital to life. Without skin we would have no protection against the elements or against other assaults from the outside such as accident, injury and infection. Even more importantly, our bodies would be unable to maintain their internal balance. In fact, it is true to say that when something goes wrong with the skin, it can have a knock-on effect on virtually every other part of the body.

The skin is made up of two layers of tissue. The outermost surface of the skin is a paper-thin waterproof layer called the epidermis, which acts as a barrier and prevents water and other fluids from being lost from the body. These surface cells are actually dead and the epidermis contains no blood vessels. This is why if you sustain a minor scratch or surface graze you may smart but you will not bleed.

Beneath the epidermis lies a much thicker, stronger layer of living tissue known as the dermis, which is made up of tough, fibrous proteins and is richly endowed with blood vessels. The main job of the dermis is to support and nourish the epidermis, and it is also closely connected to practically every other system in the body.

Underneath the dermis lies yet another layer (not strictly skin) known as the hypodermis, which consists mainly of fat and connective tissue. It is this layer that insulates our bodies against the cold and also acts as a shock absorber so that our bones and joints do not jar every time we move or reach out to touch something.

The epidermis

The epidermis is a complex structure made up of several different kinds of specialized cells, all designed to protect our

---

PROTECTION

As we have already seen, the epidermis acts as the front line between our bodies and the outside world. While it can absorb some substances such as oxygen, carbon dioxide and fat-soluble vitamins, it also repels unwelcome invaders such as bacteria, UV radiation and many other substances that could harm the body or upset its natural balance, and also protects the body against injury. It does this by the following means.

○ Keratinocytes form a physical barrier which protects the body against injury.

○ A layer of chemicals forms an 'acid mantle' over the skin's surface to repel invasion.

○ An invisible layer of sebum, an oily substance, helps kill or check the growth of bacteria and viruses.

○ Melanin shields and protects the body from the damage that can be caused by the sun.

○ Specialized immune cells help activate the body's defence mechanism – the immune system.

---

bodies and help us survive. These are arranged in several layers, or strata – as many as five in thick-skinned areas such as the soles of the feet.

Keratinocytes

By far the most plentiful cells are keratinocytes, so-called because they manufacture keratin, a tough, fibrous protein which is also present in our nails and hair. Seen under a microscope, the keratinocytes look a bit like flat crazy-paving stones. Throughout our lives they are continually dividing and moving up to the skin surface, where they die and are shed in the form of millions of tiny, virtually invisible scales. As they are shed they are replaced by new cells. These scales are of particular importance to eczema sufferers because they provide food for dust mites, which are among the most common allergens that can trigger eczema.

Keratinocytes are formed in the deepest layer of the epidermis and it takes several weeks for them to reach the surface and be shed, although in parts of our bodies which have to contend with a lot of friction, such as our hands and feet, the cycle is faster.

As we get older keratinocytes become less active and the skin's horny layer becomes thinner. This in turn leads to increased dryness and water loss, and is one reason why older people are prone to eczema craquele or asteatotic eczema, in which the skin takes on a crackled appearance.

Melanocytes

Less abundant are melanocytes, the melanin cells. These are spider-shaped cells which produce a brown pigment called melanin, a chemical our bodies produce in order to absorb ultraviolet light and protect us from sun damage. The amount of melanin in the skin determines both the skin colour and the depth to which it develops a suntan.

Melanocytes are found in the deepest layer of the epidermis. After melanin is formed it is taken up by the keratinocytes, which transport melanin to the surface where it enables the skin to withstand the effects of ultraviolet (UV) radiation from the sun. When we go to a hot country, the skin produces more melanin than it usually would in response to the sun. The melanin takes a few days to be transported to the surface of the skin, which is why it is especially important to protect yourself against the harmful effects of the sun by using a high-factor sun-protection product during the first few days spent in a hot climate.

Each one of us has the same number of melanocytes, but in dark-skinned people the melanocytes are larger and produce more melanin. Whatever the initial colour of the skin, with age it will produce less melanin and gradually become lighter.

Other cells

Other important cells found in the epidermis include Langerhans cells. These specialized cells are produced in the bone marrow and form part of the body's immune response which protects us against disease or infection. Also found in the epidermis are Merkel cells, which help us to sense touch.

The dermis

The epidermis is attached to the skin's second layer, the dermis, by means of tiny projections, or dermal papillae. These are rich in capillaries and nerve endings, enabling us to react instantly to sensations of warmth, cold, touch, pressure, irritation and pain. The wavy ridges formed by the dermal papillae can be clearly seen at our fingertips as fingerprints and on the soles of our feet.

The dermis is like a living foundation garment which holds the body together. It is made up of thick bundles of collagen – a tough, fibrous protein which gives the skin its strength and resilience and helps to keep it moist – together with another tough, yet elastic fibrous tissue called elastin which gives skin its springiness. Sometimes when skin is stretched a great deal, for example by the expanding womb in pregnancy or in sudden weight gain, the dermis is torn, which produces 'stretch marks'.

The dermis is well-endowed with blood vessels which act like mini radiators to warm the body when necessary or to help it get rid of excess heat. It is also rich in nerve fibres, which send constant messages to the brain informing it about the outside environment. The dermis is also well supplied with oil glands, sweat glands and hair follicles.

What the skin does

The skin has a variety of functions, most of which are concerned with protecting the body and helping it to maintain its natural internal balance – a process known as homeostasis.

Heat regulation

You may have wondered how the body manages to maintain a more or less constant temperature while skiing in the Alps or sunbathing on a Caribbean beach. The answer lies again, largely, in the activity of the skin. Blood vessels in the dermis regulate internal heat either by opening up (dilating) when our bodies need to rid themselves of excess heat, or closing down (constricting) to conserve heat in the body's vital internal organs when the outside temperature is cold. Dilation of the blood vessels brings more blood close to the surface of the skin where it can be cooled down by the outside air, while constriction keeps the blood in the centre of the body where it will stay warmer. When you blush or flush it is because the blood vessels close to the skin's surface have dilated, so more blood is flowing through them. By contrast, on an icy day you may notice that your skin has become very pale. This is due to the fact that the blood vessels in the skin have constricted to maintain heat inside your body.

SKIN FACTS

O Surface area: 1.5–2 sq m (1⅘–2⅖ sq yd).

O Weight: 4 kg (8¾ lb) – around 7 per cent of total body weight.

O Thickness: 1.5–4.0 mm (⅟₁₈–⅛ in).

O 1 sq cm (³⁄₂₀ sq in) of skin contains 70 cm (28 in) of blood vessels, 55 cm (22 in) of nerves, 100 sweat glands, 15 oil glands, 230 sensory receptors and 500,000 cells.

O The average person sheds 18 kg (39½ lb) of skin cells in a lifetime.

O The skin contains 5 per cent of the body's entire blood supply.

The body has another method of regulating heat: sweating. It does this by means of sweat glands which are also to be found in the dermis. As we go about our everyday lives, these glands produce small, virtually undetectable amounts of sweat. But if the heat rises, for example during exercise or hot weather, the brain receives notification of the temperature rise from nerve receptors in the skin. The brain then sends messages back via the nerves, which tell blood vessels in the dermis to widen, as we have already seen, and they also tell the sweat glands to produce more cooling sweat. If the temperature plummets, exactly the opposite happens – the blood vessels narrow and sweat production is reduced. The mechanism of sweating also helps rid the body of waste chemicals such as ammonia and urea.

Sensation

What makes a mohair sweater itch? Why do you flinch if someone pulls your hair? And what makes you pull away your hand from a burning hot plate or a sharp knife? The answer lies in special nerve receptors found in the skin. These receptors are sensitive to different types of stimuli such as pressure, temperature, pain and irritation.

Metabolic processes

The skin also plays an important role in various chemical processes that take place in the body, known as metabolic processes. Perhaps the most obvious example is the one we have already looked at: the production of melanin. However, the skin also stimulates the production of the fat-soluble vitamin D, sometimes called the 'sunshine vitamin', by reacting to sunlight on the skin. Vitamin D is needed, among other things, to enable our bodies to absorb the mineral calcium which is vital for healthy bones and teeth. This is an example of how the skin works in harmony with other body organs and tissues.

Scientists and doctors make use of this amazing ability of the skin when prescribing certain topical drugs (that is, drugs applied direct to the skin) as treatment. For instance, in conditions such as eczema, the drug cortisone is often prescribed in a topical preparation which the skin cells then change into the more powerful body hormone, hydrocortisone, which quells inflammation.

What can go wrong?

Because the skin is so closely related to the body's internal balance, when anything goes wrong with the body it often shows itself in the skin. In fact, eczema, or dermatitis, is just one of over a thousand different skin conditions and disorders. These include disorders of cell turnover, such as psoriasis, problems triggered by increased hormone production, such as acne, as well as eczema itself, which is frequently triggered by an over-sensitive immune reaction to certain factors in the environment.

Eczema disturbs virtually all the activities of the skin and this often has a knock-on effect. For example, because eczema affects the production of natural oils or sebum, the skin becomes drier and sheds more than the usual number of keratinocytes. At the same time, scratching can damage the skin's protective outer layer, causing cracks or breaks which are then prone to infection with bacteria or yeasts.

Oddly, thirst can be a symptom of eczema, because the inflammatory reaction involved in this condition causes more fluid than usual to be lost from the deeper layers of skin.

Eczema also unbalances the heat-control mechanism. Inflammation causes blood vessels within the dermis to dilate, resulting in redness and heat. As the body tries to compensate for the heat being lost through the red hot skin, blood is diverted from the internal organs causing a loss of heat and sensitivity to cold. Likewise, if you move from the cold outside to a warm room you may soon begin to feel overheated.

Under the skin

Nerves

The skin protects the nervous system. Nerve receptors in the skin enable us to sense touch. Nerve messages trigger dilation and constriction of blood vessels in the skin.

Lungs and airways

The skin protects the lungs and airways, which in turn supply skin cells with oxygen and remove carbon dioxide.

Digestive system

The skin protects the digestive organs and supplies vitamin D which is needed for the metabolism of calcium. Vitamins and minerals from digested food supply nourishment to the skin.

Muscles

The skin protects the muscles. When the muscles are working hard, heat is produced which increases blood flow and triggers sweating through the skin, helping to cool the muscles.

Immune system

The skin prevents invaders from entering the body and is involved in triggering the body's immune response.

Hormonal system

The skin protects the hormone-producing organs, and acts to convert some hormones to an active form. Sex hormones trigger the production of skin oils, for example in acne.

Heart and blood vessels

The skin protects and prevents fluid loss from the blood and acts as a reservoir for the blood supply. Oxygen and nutrients from the skin are carried in the bloodstream and waste products are disposed of through the skin.

Reproductive organs

The skin protects the reproductive organs. It also produces chemicals in sweat which attract the opposite sex. During pregnancy changes in the skin include pigmentation changes, increased sweating and sebum production. At the menopause, collagen decreases leading to loss of elasticity and thinner skin.

Urinary system

The skin protects the urinary system and rids the body of certain waste products in sweat.

Bones

The skin protects the bones. It synthesizes vitamin D which is needed for calcium absorption and strong bones. The bones act as a framework to support the skin.

2 Understanding eczema

Eczema, or dermatitis (to use a term increasingly favoured by many doctors), is one of the most common medical problems in the world. In the UK alone, one in ten people – that's one in twelve adults and one in five children – suffers from eczema and 10–20 per cent of the workload of dermatologists (doctors who specialize in the care and treatment of skin diseases) is taken up by treating people with eczema.

Alarmingly, the incidence of eczema is rising. In the last 30 years the number of people with eczema has more than doubled, a rise which can almost certainly be attributed to facets of our modern way of life, such as higher levels of pollution, central heating and food allergies.

Eczema costs a staggering £288 million every year in the UK – a third of which is spent by people with eczema themselves on bath oils, lotions, creams, ointments and other treatments. At the same time, occupational dermatitis, a type of skin inflammation caused by contact with irritant substances used in the workplace, is thought to account for over half of the working days lost in the UK every year.

What is eczema?

The word 'eczema' comes from a Greek word *ekzeein* which means to boil over. It is a description that sums up only too vividly the swelling caused by fluid accumulating in the skin which then breaks out, and the almost intolerable itching, swelling and redness that accompany this. 'Dermatitis', a term many doctors use as well as or instead of eczema, is also Greek in origin, in this case a combination of two words: *derma*, for skin, and *itis*, meaning inflammation. So dermatitis literally means 'skin inflammation'.

What's in a name?

There is a great deal of confusion about the terms eczema and dermatitis. As we have seen, both broadly mean skin inflammation. In the past the word eczema was used to distinguish skin inflammation caused by an inherited tendency to develop allergies (for example atopic eczema) from types of skin inflammation caused by other factors such as contact with external irritants (for example, contact dermatitis). Today, although you may still find these distinctions, many dermatologists prefer to use the catch-all term dermatitis for skin inflammation and to tag on a descriptive word such as 'contact' or 'atopic' to identify its cause. Other doctors use the terms eczema and dermatitis interchangeably.

Who gets eczema?

Eczema strikes people of all ages. Children are particularly prone to the most common form, atopic (allergic) eczema. In fact, one Scottish study revealed that five times as many children as adults suffered from atopic eczema. However, other types of eczema such as asteatotic and varicose eczema more commonly affect older people.

People often talk about eczema as if it were a single condition, but this is not the case. In fact, there are several different types. Some mainly affect babies and children and disappear as they reach their teens, while others are more common in adulthood or in later life – although fewer than one in fifty people aged over forty-five who develop eczema have it for the first time. A few people suffer a single attack of eczema, but many are plagued by chronic forms of the condition that can last for many years.

What effects does eczema have?

Skin symptoms such as itchiness, redness, dryness and scaling are the most well-known effects of eczema. However, there may also be other symptoms that are not obviously related to the skin. Examples include thirst, caused by loss of fluid from the skin tissues, and over-sensitivity to cold and heat, caused by the condition's effect on the body's heat-control mechanism (see page 20).

Eczema is also often associated with other allergic conditions affecting other systems of the body, in particular asthma, hay fever and rhinitis, which affect the respiratory system. And it can also render sufferers more vulnerable to a number of other medical conditions such as swollen glands, tummy aches and urinary problems (see page 35). Although eczema itself is not a life-threatening condition, some of its complications can, unless treated, pose a serious threat to health.

What causes eczema?

Many of the underlying mechanisms that cause eczema have yet to be fully understood. However, over recent years doctors have been making strides in understanding several of the key factors involved, especially in atopic eczema.

The genetic blueprint you inherit from your parents is perhaps the most important factor in atopic eczema. It is not eczema itself that you inherit but the tendency for your body to over-react to substances in your environment such as house dust mites, pollen, flakes of skin shed by household pets, feathers, fungus spores and certain foods.

Inheriting atopic genes alone is not enough to spark off eczema; it is also necessary to be exposed to certain factors in the environment. Research has shown that babies and small children who are exposed to allergens at an early age (even in the womb) are more likely to develop eczema, asthma or hay fever. What is more, the longer they are exposed to an allergen and the larger the quantity they are exposed to, the more likely they are to develop an allergy. That is why it is especially important for pregnant women and new mothers who come from atopic families, or whose partners come from atopic families, to do everything they can to avoid potential allergens (see page 29).

Having said this, exposure to allergens is not the whole story either. Intriguingly, scientists have discovered that the more colds babies and toddlers contract, the *less likely* they are to develop allergies. It is not known why this should be. However, it could be that catching infections somehow 'primes' the immune system to react in a healthy way to infections rather than being triggered by essentially harmless substances as it is in eczema.

Although the mechanisms that make someone develop eczema have yet to be fully understood, one thing is certain: once you have an allergy such as eczema, many factors in your environment can make it worse. These are known as irritants and can include cigarette smoke, alcohol, exhaust fumes, stress or emotional trauma, infections, over-exertion, overheating, over-bathing, textiles such as wool, household chemicals and cosmetics. However the key point to bear in mind is that by avoiding or curbing your exposure to such irritants you can help control your eczema.

The allergic reaction

An allergy is when your immune system reacts to a substance that is normally harmless as if it were a threat to the body, known as an allergen. Someone who has a tendency to develop allergies such as eczema, asthma and hay fever is known as 'atopic', from the Greek word *atopos* meaning out of place. The atopic tendency is usually inherited, which is why if you have eczema your parents or other family members may also have eczema or other allergic conditions such as asthma, hay fever or rhinitis. Research is going on to try to identify the gene or genes that predispose people to atopy.

When someone is atopic, his or her body produces excess amounts of the allergy antibody, a chemical called Immuno-globulin E, or IgE for short. When someone who is atopic encounters an allergen, it is IgE that sparks the immune system into action, triggering a complicated chemical chain reaction which results in the symptoms of swelling, redness and itching. The symptoms will affect different parts of the body depending on the type of condition you have. If you have eczema, the symptoms will be skin-based. With asthma, they will affect the lungs, or with hay fever, the nose and eyes.

Sensitization

An allergic reaction never takes place the first time someone encounters an allergen. The body has to learn how to react or to become sensitized to the allergen. This is what happens.

Step one The body encounters an allergen which is (wrongly) identified by blood cells in the immune system as a threat to the body.

Step two Days or sometimes weeks later the body produces allergic antibodies.

Step three The allergic antibodies attach themselves to cells in body tissues called mast cells. These mast cells release a substance called histamine which causes the symptoms of itching, redness and swelling.

Step four The next time the body encounters the same allergen, the immune system recognizes it as an enemy.

Step five The immune system swings into action, causing the symptoms of allergy.

Can eczema be prevented?

Although a genetic predisposition to allergy is unchangeable, it is your environment that pulls the trigger. Research has shown that avoiding various trigger factors could play a significant part in helping prevent children from developing allergies including eczema.

It is especially worthwhile considering ways to avoid these triggers if you or your partner have an allergic condition, although all parents and parents-to-be could benefit from following these points.

Avoiding triggers

Consider your baby's birthday Research has shown that babies born before the peak pollen season – between mid-autumn and early winter – are especially likely to become sensitized to pollen and subsequently to develop hay fever. Although the risk is small, it may be worth bearing this in mind when you are planning a pregnancy.

Think about where you live Babies living in towns and cities during the first two years of life are more likely to develop asthma and allergy. Although many of us don't have the luxury of choosing where we live, if you are in a position to choose, it may be worth considering moving to the country.

Stop smoking during pregnancy Allergic conditions, especially asthma, are more common in babies and children whose parents smoke. If you are a smoker, the most important single thing you can do for your unborn baby is to quit.

Avoid smoking indoors If you haven't managed to quit smoking, do not smoke indoors after your baby is born.

Watch out for damp Living in a damp environment can increase the likelihood of a baby or child developing an allergy – probably because house dust mites thrive in a warm, damp atmosphere. Sort out any damp problems at source or invest in a dehumidifier.

Don't overprotect your child The old adage 'You have to eat a peck of dirt before you die' has been proved to be true with regard to allergies. Children who play outside more and who develop infections in their first year of life are less likely to develop allergies.

Diet matters Various dietary measures can help reduce your child's risk of developing allergies. See Chapter 6, pages 117–119.

Types of eczema and dermatitis

Most children and adults with eczema have one of two types, atopic eczema or contact dermatitis, but there are other forms.

Atopic eczema

Atopic or allergic eczema is the most common type of eczema. It is caused by an allergic response to substances such as house dust mites, animal dander, pollen, moulds and sometimes to foods such as eggs, cows' milk, wheat, fish, chocolate, nuts, yeast and citrus fruits. It can be exacerbated by other irritants such as cigarette smoke, and emotional factors such as stress.

The severity of atopic eczema varies. For some people it may only involve the occasional patch of dry skin. However, sometimes symptoms can be severely disabling and disruptive and go on for years. Children with severe atopic eczema may face problems with lessons such as art and craft, science, design and technology and sports, while adults who have the condition may find it difficult to operate a computer, prepare food, walk, run, dance or swim.

Although atopic eczema can affect the skin on almost any area of the body, it commonly affects the head, face and neck, the arms, behind the knees and the toes.

Who gets atopic eczema?

Anyone of any age can develop atopic eczema but it strikes most often in childhood. Over six out of ten sufferers develop eczema before they are one year old and nine out of ten before they are five. The term infantile atopic eczema is used to describe atopic eczema affecting children under five. The condition rarely strikes before three months of age and usually it comes on before six months.

The first sign of atopic eczema is often a red rash on the child's cheeks, forehead and scalp. Frequently this rash becomes blistered and weepy before drying out and crusting over. The rash may spread to other areas of the skin, especially the creases of the elbows and the wrists, between the thighs and the buttocks, at the backs of the knees and ankles and behind the ears.

At this age the itching is often intolerable, causing the baby or young child to rub or scratch. Unfortunately this just makes matters worse because the skin consequently becomes broken and damaged, leading to a miserable vicious circle of itching and scratching which experts call 'the itch-scratch cycle'. The good news is that for half of those who develop eczema below the age of a year, the condition burns itself out by the age of five – with or without treatment.

In those children who are unlucky enough to continue suffering from atopic eczema or who develop it after the age of five, there is usually less weeping and crusting but more redness, dryness and lichenification (see 'symptoms of eczema' on page 35). *Keratosis pilaris*, the little bumps of keratin often found on the upper arms, is also more likely to develop in older children.

Adult atopic eczema

As we have already seen, most sufferers with infantile atopic eczema grow out of it by the time they start school, and most of those who don't wave goodbye to the condition in their teens, although it can persist until later life. It is pretty rare to develop it after the age of 30. When eczema does develop at this age, it is often brought on by harsh conditions; it mostly strikes those living in towns or cities and in climates that have low humidity.

In adults with atopic eczema, blistering and weeping are usually less troublesome. However, the leathery thickening known as lichenification is often more obvious and the skin will almost certainly be very sensitive. Sufferers will also be more prone to other allergic skin complaints such as urticaria, or nettle rash (see 'atopic eczema and other skin conditions', pages 34–5). Adults often experience dry itching skin on small areas such as the ankles, elbows, wrists or neck, although virtually any part of the body can be affected and female sufferers are often prone to eczematous skin on the nipples. Other features of adult eczema include pronounced creases under the lower eyelids and scurfy, thinning eyebrows.

Symptoms of atopic eczema

Although all the causes of eczema are still not fully understood, the symptoms are easily recognizable.

Skin inflammation A key characteristic of all types of eczema and dermatitis. It causes swelling both on the skin's surface and in the underlying tissues of the dermis (see page 15).

Itching Another key characteristic. It occurs in most types of eczema but is especially marked in atopic eczema. Itching often varies in intensity. It can be worse in winter and in the evenings. One of the problems is that itching leads to scratching, which in turn can make inflammation worse and break the skin, leaving it open to infection.

Redness Medically known as erythema, from the Greek word *erythros*, meaning red, it is caused by the widening of the blood vessels in the skin, which allows increased blood to flow to the affected area.

Blisters These are known as vesicles and are caused by the allergic reaction which increases fluid accumulation in the skin tissues. The blisters may burst and the fluid ooze onto the skin where it forms scabs.

Dry, scaly skin This may be caused directly by the eczema or it may be the sufferer's natural skin type. Dry skin can occasionally predispose a person to the development of eczema and dermatitis.

Pallid skin and loss of pigmentation Because of reduced blood flow caused by eczema's disruptive effect on the skin's circulation, many children are pale in areas not affected by eczema. Eczema also disturbs the skin's production of the brown pigment melanin (see page 14), resulting in the development of pale patches of depigmented skin.

Whitening on pressure Atopic eczema affects the skin's heat-control mechanism and with it the activity of blood vessels in the skin. In around seven out of ten people with the condition, the blood vessels in the skin contract when pressure is applied to the skin, causing whitening. The condition doesn't just affect eczematous parts of the skin.

Thickened skin Over time, scratching and rubbing cause the skin to try to protect itself by producing more keratin (the tough protective protein found in skin cells). This keratinization, as it is known, leads to the development of lichenification, a medical term doctors use to describe scaly, leathery and thickened skin in which the normal skin furrows appear exaggerated.

Nail damage When the fingers are eczematous, the cuticle may be damaged, breaking the bond between the nail plate and the cuticle, which leaves the nail vulnerable to infection. This in turn can damage the surface of the nail. Other problems can be caused by skin debris getting under the nail and causing infection, due to scratching. Keeping the nails short should help avert this.

Eye creases and 'shiners' Children with eczema often have one or two extra creases in the skin beneath the eyes which may have a bluish tinge, commonly known as 'shiners'. They are probably due to swelling caused by an eczematous reaction below the eye, although the reason why these creases have a bluish tinge is not clear.

Atopic eczema and other skin conditions

People with atopic eczema often have sensitive skin generally and can be prone to other skin conditions such as urticaria, also known as hives, or nettle rash or psoriasis. People with urticaria develop inflammation with itchy, raised, white or yellow weals, which may merge to form large, irregular patches on the limbs or the trunk. It happens when the person is exposed to an offending substance – often foods such as milk, eggs, strawberries, nuts or shellfish. The food triggers a chain reaction in which the chemical histamine is released from the skin cells, causing fluid to seep into the tissue. It is this that causes the subcutaneous skin swelling which is visible as weals. Contrary to popular opinion, people with eczema can have psoriasis as well. The condition, which causes thickened patches of inflamed, red skin covered in silvery scales, is a result of an acceleration of the normal turnover of skin cells. This causes live keratinocytes to accumulate on the surface of the skin where they form the typical thickened patches with silvery scales. Unlike eczema, psoriasis does not cause itching. Psoriasis and eczema do not often occur together, however.

Associated medical problems

If your child has eczema, often, though not always, he or she may be vulnerable to certain other medical problems. These may include:

Asthma and hay fever Children with atopic eczema are prone to other allergic conditions, in particular asthma and hay fever.

Poor growth Children with atopic eczema may be smaller than usual for their age. Although the mechanism responsible is not understood, when the eczema is treated, the child often has a surge of growth and catches up with other children of the same age.

Runny nose Children with atopic eczema are often prone to a condition known as allergic rhinitis, which produces cold-like symptoms. It is caused by an allergic reaction to airborne allergens such as dust, mould and animal dander.

Swollen glands Children with eczema often experience swollen glands in the neck, the armpits and groin. The so-called 'glands' are in fact lymph nodes, whose job it is to protect the body against infection. In eczema they have to work harder to drain lymphatic fluid from the affected skin.

Therefore, although worrying, swollen glands are in fact a sign that the child's body is working to protect the internal organs against infection.

Tummy aches Children with eczema often complain of abdominal pain and their abdomens may stick out. Although it is not known exactly why this happens, some specialists ascribe it to 'intestinal eczema', a condition that may be linked to food allergies.

Urinary problems The urethra, the tube down which urine passes from the bladder, can become inflamed as a result of eczema, leading to soreness and burning on passing urine. This may be confused with cystitis. The doctor can prescribe treatment to cure the problem.

Anaphylactic shock This is an extreme – and sometimes fatal – allergic reaction that can be triggered by an insect sting, an injection or the consumption of certain foods, such as prawns or peanuts.

The immune system over-reacts to these triggers, causing dizziness, headache, a tight chest, swollen eyelids and lips and difficulty breathing. It is vital that immediate treatment with an adrenalin injection or inhaler is given. If you are present when this happens, lie the child down with raised knees and call an ambulance, or take him or her to hospital. If you believe your child is at risk, ask your doctor if your child should wear a MedicAlert bracelet.

Contact dermatitis

The second main type of eczema is known as contact dermatitis, a term used to describe skin irritation caused, literally, by contact with an external substance. There are two main types of this condition: irritant contact dermatitis, sometimes known as 'wear and tear' dermatitis, and allergic contact dermatitis.

Irritant contact dermatitis

Unlike atopic eczema or dermatitis, irritant contact dermatitis is not linked to an allergic reaction. It is a skin reaction caused by irritating chemicals such as detergents, bleaches, paint, cement, fertilizers and even soil and water. These chemicals strip away the skin's natural oils (sebum) causing the skin to become red, dry and itchy. Left untreated, the condition may become persistent (chronic) and the skin may crack, causing a risk of infection.

The condition can strike anyone, but it is most common in people whose jobs or everyday lives involve repeated contact with strong, irritating substances. Such people include nurses, hairdressers, cleaners, farm-workers, painters and decorators, builders and rubber and textile workers. Having said that, almost any substance can cause problems, including household chemicals like washing-up liquid, and foods such as cheese, citrus fruits, onions, garlic, radishes and tomatoes.

Allergic contact dermatitis

Like atopic eczema, allergic contact dermatitis is caused by an allergic reaction, only in this case the reaction occurs as a result of direct skin contact between the allergen and the skin. The condition can strike at any time and is extremely common: an estimated two in one hundred Westerners are affected. Like irritant contact dermatitis, it is especially common among people who use chemicals at work.

Symptoms of redness, inflammation, open sores and scabbing appear on the area of skin exposed to the substance – usually some 1–3 days after contact with the offending chemical. Sometimes a secondary rash appears elsewhere on the skin. Commonly affected areas include the face and neck, under the arms, the arms, trunk, thighs, calves and the feet.

If you are not sure whether you have irritant contact dermatitis or allergic contact dermatitis, bear in mind that an allergic reaction never appears on the first contact with an allergen, but on the second or subsequent exposure. This is because the immune system which produces the allergic reaction basically has to be 'primed' before it releases antibodies.

Common allergens in allergic contact dermatitis are:

❑ metals such as nickel and cobalt used in jewellery, zips and studs;
❑ perfumes found in soaps, cosmetics and toiletries;
❑ preservatives used in cosmetics and toiletries such as face and hand creams;
❑ hair dyes and dyes found in clothing and shoes;
❑ lanolin used in cosmetics and toiletries
❑ rubber used to make rubber gloves, boots, shoes, condoms and other goods;
❑ chromate, a chemical used in tanned leather, matches and cement
❑ plants such as primulas, chrysanthemums, ivy and tulips.

Other types of dermatitis

There are hundreds of other skin disorders that involve skin inflammation, and some of the most common are listed here.

Many can be alleviated by the self-help methods outlined in Chapter 3, pages 45–63. However, if you think you or your child has one of them, it is important to consult your doctor to get a proper diagnosis.

Vesicular (pompholyx) eczema or dermatitis

This condition, which is often a complication of atopic eczema or contact dermatitis, causes itchy blisters, or vesicles, to appear on the sides of the fingers, palms of the hands and soles of the feet. These may burst and become infected. Alternatively, the skin may dry out and peel or crack. The condition is often worse in warm weather as it is aggravated by heat and sweating.

Seborrhoeic eczema or dermatitis

This is a skin disorder that tends to begin with itching and scaliness on the scalp, causing severe dandruff. This may spread to the face and, in particular, oily zones such as the sides of the nose, eyebrows, ears, the margin of the scalp and upper body. Sufferers may be especially sensitive to chemicals in products such as soaps, bubble baths and cosmetics.

Infantile seborrhoeic eczema, otherwise known as 'cradle cap', strikes babies during their first year of life. As well as on the scalp, the baby may develop red, scaly patches, similar in appearance to atopic eczema, in areas where the skin rubs together, for example at the elbows or under the armpits. However, unlike atopic eczema there is little itching and lichenification does not occur. Although unsightly, the condition tends to disappear of its own accord around the age of nine months.

Nummular or discoid eczema

People who had atopic eczema as a baby sometimes develop nummular or discoid eczema as adults. The term 'nummular', which comes from the Latin *nummus,* meaning small coin, describes the small, scaly, slightly swollen, coin-shaped patches that develop and sometimes blister and weep before crusting over. The patches, which can be itchy, are most often found on the backs of the hands and legs in a symmetrical pattern. The biggest risk is that they may get infected. It may be triggered by the skin becoming dry, especially in winter or in conditions of low humidity.

Light-sensitive eczema

Light-sensitive eczema, otherwise known as photosensitive or chronic actinic eczema, is a kind of eczema that appears after exposure to the sun. The culprits are the ultraviolet (UV) rays emitted by the sun. The condition usually affects men more than women and, not surprisingly, is often worse in the spring and summer, although because ultraviolet rays can penetrate cloud, it can also develop in less sunny seasons of the year. If you already have another form of eczema or dermatitis it can be made worse by light sensitivity.

The rash, which is itchy and red, may become sore and weepy. Although it is most often visible on areas of the skin left bare, such as the backs of the hands, forearms and face, it may also spread to other areas of skin that haven't been exposed to sunlight. The condition can sometimes be triggered by the use of drugs and other chemicals that interact with sunlight, such as some anti-histamine drugs and anti-bacterial substances found in certain toiletries.

Lichen simplex

A patch or patches of thickened, itchy and possibly discoloured skin on the neck, wrist, arms, ankles or in the genital area may signal a type of eczema known as lichen simplex or neurodermatitis. It affects more women than men and is caused by the repeated rubbing or scratching of a patch of skin, sometimes almost unconsciously as a result of anxiety or stress. This leads to a vicious cycle of scratching and itching.

Varicose eczema

Also known as stasis or gravitational eczema, this usually occurs in middle-aged to older people who have had varicose veins or a deep-vein thrombosis. Women and overweight people are more at risk. The skin of the lower legs and ankles becomes blotchy, inflamed, swollen, itchy and discoloured as a result of poor circulation in the lower legs caused by weakness or damage to the valves of the leg veins. The skin tends to be thin due to a lack of nutrients, and may split and form a varicose ulcer.

Asteatotic eczema

Although increased skin dryness and thinning is a normal part of the ageing process, in asteatotic eczema, or eczema craquele, the skin is stripped of its natural oils, giving it a crackled appearance a bit like an antique vase. It usually appears first on the fronts of the lower legs.

Possible complications of eczema

The skin of eczema sufferers is more vulnerable to infections than non-sufferers. This is because eczema may breach the skin's protective mantle, causing open wounds where micro-organisms such as bacteria, viruses and fungi can thrive. Also, because eczema damages all the skin's functions including its immune response (see Chapter 1, pages 19–21), it is unable to fight off outside enemies so effectively.

A wide number of different micro-organisms can affect the skin. Of these, by far the most serious is the herpes simplex virus. This can cause a type of eczema known as eczema herpeticum, or Kaposi's varicelliform eruption (this has no connection with the well-known Kaposi's sarcoma caused by AIDS). Kaposi's varicelliform eruption can also be caused by the *Staphylococcus aureus* bacterium.

For this reason, it is important for anyone with eczema to keep well away from anyone with cold sores, which are caused by the herpes simplex virus. You should never kiss anyone with a cold sore as there is a risk of contracting a serious, widespread infection that may spread to the brain and the spinal cord. If you or your child have been in contact with anyone with a cold sore, it is vital to see the doctor so that an anti-viral drug can be prescribed.

Other germs that can infect eczematous skin include the wart virus HPV (human papillomavirus), fungi (including those that cause athlete's foot and ringworm) and molluscum contagiosum, a virus that causes shiny, white lumps or papules to appear on the skin surface.

Living with eczema

The various complications can be daunting. They are included to arm you with information, which is one of your most important allies in your fight to control eczema. However, it is important to remember that you are highly unlikely to experience more than one or two of the different types of eczema and that most of the complications outlined are extremely rare.

Eczema or dermatitis does respond to treatment and there are many things you can do yourself to keep your skin healthy. There is no 'cure' for eczema, but with optimum medical treatment and care, plus a sensible programme of skin care, lifestyle and diet, it can usually be controlled.

3 Controlling the symptoms

The effects of eczema can be wide-ranging, but you don't have to let the condition rule your life – provided you learn how to manage it. It may seem a nuisance always to have to be thinking about your skin, but if you incorporate a sensible skin care routine into your daily life, eventually it will be no more of a burden than cleaning your teeth or brushing your hair each day.

Seeking medical treatment can help, of course, and the various medications that are available can do an enormous amount to ease symptoms during flare-ups of eczema. We will be looking in depth at these in Chapter 4. But meanwhile, there is a host of things you can do in your everyday life to protect your skin from being susceptible to eczema outbreaks and to keep it as healthy as possible.

The advice that follows in this chapter is geared towards atopic eczema, but the skin-care basics equally apply to other types of eczema and dermatitis.

Skin care – the basics

Healthy skin is perfectly designed to withstand external attack. However, when you have eczema your skin's ability to protect you is reduced, making the skin more sensitive and vulnerable. For this reason you need to take special care to keep it clean, to combat dryness, quell inflammation and itching and reduce the risk of infections.

If you suspect you or your child have eczema or dermatitis, it is important to get a proper medical diagnosis first. Medical treatment may be necessary from time to time when the condition is active to bring symptoms under control. Also, if you need to use large quantities of moisturizer it may be cheaper to get them on prescription. However, most of the steps you need to take are things you can do yourself.

Moisturize your skin

Because eczema damages the epidermis and affects the skin's production of sebum (the moisturizing natural oils that keep it supple), the most fundamental measure you can take to protect your skin is to keep it hydrated or moisturized. This means that from now on you need to get into the habit of using products called emollients, oil- or fat-based moisturizing and softening agents, on a daily basis to counteract dryness and keep your skin soft and supple.

Emollients work in two ways. Firstly, they form a protective waterproof barrier over the surface of the skin, which helps to

TIPS ON USING AN EMOLLIENT

○ Always wash your hands before applying, in order to reduce the risk of infection.

○ Apply immediately after drying your skin following a wash or bath – experts say within three minutes – to restore moisture and prevent the skin drying out.

○ Apply an emollient by dabbing on the skin before smoothing in gently.

○ Apply in the direction of hair growth and avoid over-zealous rubbing as this can spark a bout of itching.

○ Tubes or pump dispensers are handy and less likely to become contaminated by germs from your fingers.

○ Don't share your emollient with anyone else, in order to avoid cross-contamination.

keep moisture in and prevents it from being lost. Secondly they help 'stick' the surface skin cells together much in the way the skin's own natural oils do, so your skin will feel smoother and more comfortable.

Choosing an emollient

Emollients are widely available over the counter at the pharmacy or on prescription. Choosing an emollient can be difficult because they come in a huge range of different forms – creams, lotions, ointments and bath or shower products – and have a wide range of different ingredients. However, once you know what is on offer, you will be in a better position to pick the product or products that are most suitable for you.

Broadly speaking, there are two main types of emollient. These are oil-in-water emulsions or water-in-oil emulsions. Water-in-oil emulsions are heavier, more oily and tend to adhere to the skin better. But they can feel greasy and most of the time you may prefer the lighter, more absorbent oil-in-water type emulsions, which tend to be less greasy. There is another type of product that has recently emerged which is 'oil free'. However, because many of these contain silicones, they don't suit everybody.

Because people with eczema tend to have sensitive skin generally, when looking for a product it is best to check the label to make sure it contains as few additives, such as perfumes, preservatives and colourings, as possible. It is also sensible to avoid anything with lanolin (an animal fat derived from sheep's wool) as some forms of it often trigger an allergic reaction in people prone to eczema.

When first using a new product, do a patch test before applying it widely. Smooth on a small amount of the product and leave it for several hours or up to a day to check your skin does not react badly. The pharmacist can give you advice on suitable products to try. Alternatively, you can ask your doctor for a prescription, although he or she may have a favourite product that won't necessarily be the best one for you.

You will probably find that you need to obtain a number of different products for different purposes, depending on how dry your skin is and your lifestyle. For instance, at times when your skin is weepy, a cream may be the most soothing. If, on the other hand, your skin is extremely dry, you will probably find an ointment or rich cream more soothing than a lotion, which tends to be thinner and less moisturizing. However, if you are living a busy life you will probably find lotions better for times when you are in a hurry because, being thinner and less viscous, they glide on to the skin more easily. A little experimentation may be necessary to find the ones that suit you best in different circumstances.

Sample daily moisturizing regimen

8 am   Bath or shower using an emollient oil. Apply moisturizing cream to the whole of your body.

11 am–11 pm Apply moisturizing lotion as needed, especially to your hands.

11 pm   Apply moisturizing ointment to the whole of your body before bed, in order to moisturize the skin overnight.

Avoiding irritants

An irritant is anything you come into contact with that irritates your skin. Common culprits include wool or synthetic fibres found in clothing or furniture, perfumes and cosmetics, chemicals such as chlorine found in swimming pools, bleach, mineral oils or solvents, dust, sand and cigarette smoke.

You may find that soap is a particular problem because it dries out the skin and strips it of its natural oils. Many soaps also contain perfume which can trigger an allergic reaction. You'll probably find it is better to use a soap substitute, such as a cleansing bar, skin wash or cream, specially designed for dry, sensitive skin. Other alternatives include two products available from the pharmacy known as emulsifying ointment and aqueous cream – a mixture of emulsifying ointment, an agent called phenoxyethanol and water. You can use them just like soap but they are less harsh on the skin.

Avoid excessive water

As you have probably found out through bitter experience, too much bathing, swimming or showering can leach away moisture and strip the skin of its natural oils, making it drier, itchier and more sensitive. Although it is important to keep the skin clean, you should do your best to limit your exposure to water, especially hard water, and products such as bubble baths, bath salts and other preparations. Avoid prolonged bathing or showering – no longer than ten minutes – and consider having a water softener attached to the bath or shower taps.

Going swimming can be troublesome because as well as the adverse effects of being immersed in water, the chlorine used to disinfect the water can also be irritating. However, it is a pity to miss out on the fun and benefits of the exercise. To prevent the skin from drying out when swimming, apply a thick barrier such as petroleum jelly, then shower well afterwards and apply an emollient.

Treat your skin gently

If you are prone to eczema or dermatitis, you must treat your skin gently at all times. When having a bath or shower, use lukewarm water as hot water can cause redness and itching. Whatever you do, you should steer well clear of harsh exfoliating scrubs and products containing fruit acids (Alpha Hydroxy Acids or AHAs). You should also avoid any kind of vigorous towelling or exfoliating treatments such as skin brushing. When drying your skin, it is best to gently dab it dry with a soft towel, and when you are applying a moisturizing cream you should do so gently.

Protect your hands

So many jobs around the house involve immersing the hands in water, so it's not surprising that the hands of eczema sufferers are especially prone to dryness and cracking. Whatever kind of eczema or dermatitis you have, it is important to protect your hands. Invest in some cotton-lined waterproof gloves to wear when doing jobs like washing or cleaning, and wear a pair of plain cotton gloves for other household tasks such as dusting and vacuuming.

Watch what you wear

If you have eczema, the fabric you put next to your skin can make all the difference between a comfortable skin and a hot, irritated one that is crying out to be scratched. Both wool and synthetic fibres can be problematic, as can rough or badly fitting clothes. Cotton and cotton mixes are usually the best bet and you should avoid wearing tight, constricting clothes which will make you hot and sweaty.

When you go shopping for clothes, be sure to check labels to find out what they are made from, and wash any clothes before you wear them to remove potentially irritant finishes or excess dyes. Although you will usually be able to tell if a garment is irritating when you try it on, you should pay special attention to seams and zips, which often contain nickel (a common culprit in contact eczema).

Pay special attention to tights and socks – again, it is best to go for cotton or a cotton mix. Try to avoid wearing the same shoes every day to prevent moisture build-up. During the winter months, it is best to wear long cotton underwear with layers on top for warmth.

Stay cool

Many types of eczema, including atopic eczema and vesicular eczema, are aggravated by heat and sweating, so it is important to keep your body as cool as possible, especially in hot weather. Wearing loose cotton clothing will help and you should also make every effort to keep your house cool and well ventilated. The bedroom, especially, should be kept cool – ideally below 16°C (61°F).

In winter, don't sit close to an open fire or radiator, and make sure the central heating is not turned up too high. Central heating can also dry out the air, which can in turn dry out the skin and make itching more troublesome. Try to keep the air moist by using a humidifier or placing bowls of water around the house.

Having said all this, extreme cold can also irritate the skin, so wrap up warm before going out in winter and protect exposed skin with a layer of petroleum jelly.

Identifying and eliminating triggers

Although dermatologists do not understand exactly why some people develop atopic eczema, they do know that certain allergens or triggers often spark off an attack. Triggers are not the cause of eczema because the tendency to develop the condition is inborn, but as the name suggests they can prompt a flare-up (see pages 29–30). Research suggests that the time in life when you are exposed to an allergen and the amount to which you are exposed are the key factors in determining your reaction to it.

As well as the specific skin irritants already mentioned, there are several well-known common triggers for eczema, asthma and hay fever. Their effect varies from one person to another and to a certain extent from one occasion to another. Unless you are very unlucky, you are unlikely to be affected by all of them. You may find you can enter a house with a cat one day and it has no effect, but another day it sparks off an attack of eczema. Getting to know your personal triggers and doing all you can to minimize contact with them can dramatically improve the health of your skin and therefore reduce your chances of suffering a flare-up of eczema.

Pollen

Although pollen is more usually associated with allergic conditions affecting the respiratory system, such as asthma and hay fever, it can also spark off an eczema flare-up. Tips on avoiding pollen include:

❏ Check pollen forecasts daily on radio, television or the Internet, and try to spend as little time as possible outside on days when the count is high. If you have been outside, change your clothes when you come in and have a shower to rid yourself of specks of pollen.

❏ In seasons when the pollen count is high (mid-spring to early summer for tree pollens and throughout summer for grass pollens), keep the windows shut.

❏ Think about doing away with the lawn. Perhaps have a Japanese-style garden with pebbles and paving stones instead. If you really cannot do without your patch of grass, get someone else to cut it and stay indoors with the windows shut while they are doing it.

❏ Check out the different varieties of allergen-producing plants and avoid having them in your garden.

House dust mites

The house dust mite is the most common trigger for many allergic conditions. No matter how clean it is, your house is teeming with literally millions of these microscopic insects, which survive by feeding on dead human skin cells present in house dust. They thrive in the warm, humid atmosphere of centrally heated homes, especially in carpets, mattresses, sofas and soft furnishings. It is not actually the mites themselves that trigger allergic reactions, but a protein found in their excreta. It is impossible to eradicate house dust mites entirely from your home, but you can reduce their numbers if you follow this advice:

Choose hard floors Carpets provide a wonderful home for house dust mites, especially in the bedroom. Fortunately, today there is a huge range of attractive hard flooring which is durable and easy to clean. Check out wood, cork, concrete, tiles, vinyl or newly fashionable linoleum.

Mattresses House dust mites also thrive in mattresses. Special, easy-to-clean mattress-protectors are available in department stores and bedding shops, and also by mail order. If you are buying a new mattress, get one with an in-built interliner. Foam mattresses are preferable to the interior-sprung type, which provides more places for the dust mites to breed.

Avoid feather cushions and duvets Change bedlinen at least once a week and wash at a high temperature. Air pillows, duvets and mattresses in the open to kill off mites (sunlight kills them) – but not in spring or summer when the pollen count is high.

Furnishings Blinds are preferable to curtains as they are easier to keep clean, although avoid Venetian blinds which gather dust. Soft furnishings are more likely to harbour dust. If you must have upholstered furniture, choose ones with removable covers and wash them regularly. Avoid padded headboards and choose a bed frame with a slatted base rather than a divan base. Beds and upholstered furniture can be heat treated to rid them of house dust mites.

Cleaning matters Vacuuming is preferable to sweeping as this stirs up the dust. There are several models of vacuum cleaner with special filters designed for people with dust allergies. Even so, you may find it helps to wear a mask when you are cleaning. You should also dust regularly with a damp cloth as dry dusting will scatter dust mite droppings around the room.

Check your heating Warm air duct central heating, blow heaters and convector heaters blow dust around, so if you are moving house avoid buying anywhere that has these heating systems. If you already have them, try to replace them if you can possibly afford it.

Household pets

Contact with furry animals is another major trigger factor in allergies. In fact, research suggests that exposure to pets may be a factor in as many as two out of five cases of childhood asthma. Although no such studies have been done on eczema, it is a fair guess that a similar proportion may be affected. The animal's dander, the word used to describe flakes of skin (hence dandruff), is the main allergen, but fur, dried saliva, urine and faeces can also be allergenic. Again, it is the protein in these substances that sparks off the allergic reaction.

Unfortunately, if you or a member of your family has severe eczema (or if you come from an atopic family and are planning to have a baby), to have a pet is probably a bad idea. If your eczema is less severe, you will need to think carefully about owning a pet – perhaps choosing one that does not shed dander, such as a goldfish. If you must have a cat or dog, keep it outside or instead get an animal that does not have free range of the house, such as a hamster or guinea pig. If you really can't do without a pet, you may just have to learn to live with the fact that you will need to use more medication for your eczema to compensate.

Food

Certain foods can be a problem for some children and adults, triggering a flare-up of eczema or aggravating existing symptoms. Much of this book is devoted to finding food solutions for your eczema. You will find details in Chapters 6 and 7, pages 99–170.

Thoughts, feelings and emotions

Many people with atopic eczema notice a definite link between their thoughts, emotions and feelings and their eczema. An exam, an argument with a partner, a difficult patch at work, tiredness or even a happy but stressful event such as getting married or having a baby may all spark an attack or make existing symptoms worse.

Studies show that the way we think and feel can affect the immune system, which is over-active in people suffering from eczema. When you are stressed, your body gets ready to 'fight or flight', releasing hormones such as adrenaline and cortisol, produced by the adrenal glands to speed up breathing, increase the heart rate and generally make you alert in the face of danger. The problem is that these hormones also act on the immune system, making it less effective. And because your body is on red alert when you are stressed, you are also likely to be more aware of symptoms such as soreness and itching and an increased temptation to scratch.

Stress is a simple fact of life. You cannot escape it. However, you can learn to deal with it. Making time for yourself and doing something you enjoy will help you feel less stressed, as can learning specific stress-busting techniques such as relaxation, yoga, meditation, hypnosis and positive-thinking techniques. See Chapter 5, pages 77–98, for details.

Keeping a trigger diary

One of the most helpful things you can do if you haven't already worked out the things that trigger your eczema is to keep a trigger diary. This is a daily record designed to help you to identify the specific factors that spark off your eczema. Of course you will probably already be aware of at least some of these. However, you may well find that you do not always react to them. Keeping a diary will help you to determine more precisely what factors or combination of factors are needed to spark off a flare-up.

Invest in a small notebook or diary that will fit into your bag or briefcase and carry it with you at all times. Use it to note down any potential triggers you have encountered – you may find it helpful to use the list on page 58 to jog your memory. If you are a woman, you should also keep a note of your reproductive cycle; premenstrual symptoms (PMS), pregnancy or menopausal symptoms can often be associated with flare-ups. You should also note any illnesses and any

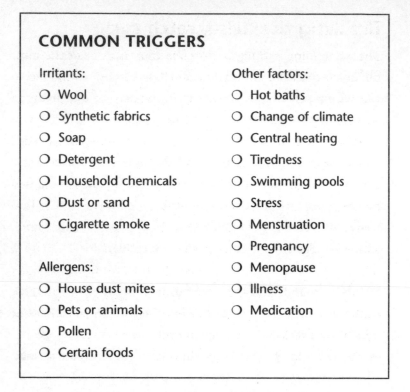

COMMON TRIGGERS

Irritants:

- O Wool
- O Synthetic fabrics
- O Soap
- O Detergent
- O Household chemicals
- O Dust or sand
- O Cigarette smoke

Allergens:

- O House dust mites
- O Pets or animals
- O Pollen
- O Certain foods

Other factors:

- O Hot baths
- O Change of climate
- O Central heating
- O Tiredness
- O Swimming pools
- O Stress
- O Menstruation
- O Pregnancy
- O Menopause
- O Illness
- O Medication

medication you take, including over-the-counter drugs, herbal or nutritional supplements and the contraceptive pill or hormone replacement therapy (HRT). Also make a note of the details of any eczema symptoms, where they are and their severity. After a while you should have enough information to enable you to trace the specific factors that worsen symptoms, bearing in mind that attacks may not come on immediately.

You can then work out a plan of action to avoid or minimize your exposure to the culprits. Of course, there are likely to be some triggers over which you have little or no control, but at least you can be prepared for an attack and take steps to alleviate symptoms and reduce its severity.

Breaking the itch-scratch cycle

The maddening itching that eczema causes is one of the most difficult aspects of the condition. It is totally instinctive to want to scratch an itch. However, if you have eczema, giving in to this urge is actually counter-productive: you itch, you scratch, you itch more. Scratching puts the nerves on edge making you itch even more – and so it goes on. In fact, a few experts even go so far as to argue that eczema is actually caused by having a 'low-itch threshold' and that it is scratching that triggers the eczematous rash rather than the other way round. Although most dermatologists do not hold this view, there is no doubt that scratching can damage the skin, leaving it open to infection and, over time, lead to lichenification – the thick leatheriness associated with eczema. The good news is that it is possible to break the itch-scratch cycle, as follows.

❏ Pay attention to the basic skin care steps which are set out on pages 47–9.

❏ Keep your skin well moisturized by applying an emollient at least twice a day and more often on your hands.

❏ Use any medication prescribed by your doctor. Antihistamine medication can help alleviate itching.

❏ Try to identify any triggers that aggravate your rash.

❏ Keep your fingernails short and wear cotton gloves in bed if necessary to prevent yourself scratching in your sleep.

❏ Try to identify patterns to your scratching. If necessary keep a diary (see page 57) to detect the times of the day or situations when you are more itchy.

❏ Check out whether there is something that is causing you to itch more, for instance synthetic bedclothes or an overheated, dry atmosphere in the bedroom.

- Try to distract yourself with an alternative activity when you feel the urge to scratch, for example reading a book, phoning a friend or dancing around your living room.
- If the urge to scratch is becoming irresistible, try rubbing instead, press on the area or apply a moisturizer or something cool such as an ice pack.
- If you absolutely must scratch, give yourself a time limit.

Helping a child with eczema

If your child has atopic eczema, you are not alone. Around one in eight children develop eczema at some time during their childhood, and it is estimated that an average school classroom will have between one and five children with eczema.

The good news is that young children do frequently grow out of their eczema. In fact, if your child developed infantile atopic eczema (see page 31) as a baby, there is an odds-on chance that he or she will be free of it by the time he or she starts school. The bad news is that for some children – often those with the most severe types of eczema – the condition does persist and virtually everyone who has ever had atopic eczema tends to have a more sensitive skin than other people without the condition.

One of the worst aspects of childhood eczema is the stress that it can cause, not just for the child who is affected, but for the whole family. When a child has any kind of chronic condition, it is natural for a parent to want to protect the child. This can sometimes lead to parents spoiling the eczematous child and paying them more attention than their other children – with predictable results on family dynamics. Although there will obviously be times when your child needs more attention, it is very important to make every effort to treat him or her in the same way as the other children and to resist the urge to over-protect, preventing the child from enjoying a normal childhood. Include your child in normal everyday family activities and don't let him or her use eczema as an excuse to avoid doing things, such as taking part in school trips or visits.

Managing a child's eczema

Much of the practical advice already outlined on how to avoid irritants and look after the skin applies equally to children as adults. Naturally, while a child is small you will have to take responsibility for his or her bathing and moisturizing routines. However, as the child grows older you can teach him or her how to measure out bath solutions and apply moisturizers and share in the self-care regime. Your child will gain confidence from knowing that he or she can control symptoms.

Because eczema is such a visible condition, it can sometimes arouse cruel remarks from other children or their parents and, in some cases, may even result in bullying. Although these comments may be the result of ignorance, they are no less hurtful for that. As always, knowledge is power. Therefore, as soon as your child is old enough, you should explain in simple terms what eczema is so that he or she can counter any negative comments. There are various picture books available that explain eczema in simple terms, which can aid you and help your child to understand his or her own condition. If the child becomes the victim of more sustained bullying or taunting, it is vital that you report it to a teacher and work out a strategy for dealing with it before it becomes entrenched.

When your child starts school, make sure that the staff are fully informed. The child will need to have access to medications and you should explain how to cope if he or she has an attack of itching. Also explain that the child may occasionally miss school because of a flare-up and that itching or tiredness may cause a lack of concentration. It is also vital that they know the dangers of the child coming into contact with children with infections such as impetigo or cold sores (see page 42).

HELPING YOUR CHILD AVOID IRRITANTS AT SCHOOL

Irritant	Action
Soap and water	Pack a special soap bar or cleanser and a soft cotton towel to use at school.
Overheating	Overheating can trigger symptoms – ask for the child to sit in a cool part of the classroom well away from radiators and windows.
Water play	The teacher should know that water can exacerbate eczema. Special vinyl gloves can be worn for water play.
Swimming	Swimming can be problematic. Applying a barrier ointment before going swimming can help. Make sure the teacher knows your child needs enough time to shower after swimming and to apply moisturizing creams and lotions.
Sports	Sports can be difficult because of embarrassment, and overheating can provoke symptoms. However, most of the time your child will benefit from exercise, so should be encouraged to take part in lessons. Make sure the sports teacher knows about your child's condition and allows time to wash and apply moisturizers after exercise.
Foods	Cookery lessons can be problematic if the child's skin is irritated by certain foods. Oranges, lemons, tomatoes, onions and spices are particular culprits. Make sure the cookery teacher is aware of this. Again, the child may need to wear gloves.
Chemicals	Your child should wear protective clothing and gloves during science lessons.

4 Orthodox medical treatment

Although most of the time you will probably be able to keep your eczema reasonably well controlled by following the self-help tips outlined in the previous chapter, however well you manage there will be times when you need the help of your doctor for diagnosis and treatment.

It is important to seek medical advice when the eczema appears for the first time so that your condition can be diagnosed. The doctor can then prescribe any suitable medication and offer advice on the various ways to alleviate the symptoms of eczema.

It is also wise to visit the doctor if the rash is spreading or seems to be getting much worse, despite self-help treatment, or if the itching and scratching become uncontrollable. You should also seek medical help if you develop a skin infection –

the signs are redness, soreness, swelling or pus – as you will need supplementary medication to combat the infection and prevent it spreading.

Tailoring the treatment to you

Just as the symptoms of eczema and dermatitis can range from mild to severe, so there is a whole spectrum of medical treatments available. Some of these can be bought over the counter at a pharmacist, others are powerful drugs which are only available on prescription from a doctor. Medication can help to relieve inflammation and itching and prevent further damage to the skin during flare-ups. With appropriate medical treatment, you can expect the condition to be brought under control within about three weeks and, although the eczema may never be totally cured, the treatment can help you to maintain better control.

Because no two people with eczema are the same, any treatment the doctor recommends should ideally be tailored to you as an individual. There are several distinct forms of treatment that may play a part in an overall treatment plan. These include: emollient therapy, corticosteroids, antibiotics and antiseptics, anti-histamines, bandages and wraps, immunosuppressive drugs, tar preparations and ultraviolet treatment (light therapy).

Emollient therapy

The importance of keeping the skin clean and well moisturized cannot be over-emphasized. For further details of the wide range of moisturizing and emollient treatments on offer, both from a pharmacist or on prescription, see Chapter 3, pages 46–49.

Corticosteroids

One of the primary aims of treating eczema is to quell the inflammatory reaction that is causing the skin symptoms. Corticosteroids – often known simply as steroids or glucocorticoids – are among the most effective and treatments. These drugs are similar to cortisol, a natural hormone produced by the body's adrenal glands. They act in two ways: firstly, by interfering with the body's ability to make the chemicals that cause inflammation, and secondly, by suppressing the activity of the immune system. Although they share the same name, the steroids used to treat eczema are not to be confused with the steroids – known as anabolic steroids – that some sportspeople take to build muscle and enhance performance.

SAFE STEROID USE

Over-the-counter hydrocortisone preparations are effective to help control mild to moderate eczema. They are perfectly safe provided you observe the following precautions during use:

○ Do read the instructions and follow them to the letter (if in doubt ask your pharmacist or doctor for advice).

○ Do apply the product thinly.

○ Do seek the advice of a doctor before using any steroid preparation if the sufferer is a pregnant woman or a child under ten.

○ Don't use the preparation more than twice a day for up to seven days.

○ Don't use it on broken or infected skin.

Corticosteroids come in different strengths and in different forms. They can either be taken by mouth (oral steroids) or applied direct to the skin (topical steroids).

Oral steroids

When steroids first became available some 50 years ago, they were hailed as wonder drugs that would revolutionize the treatment of a number of diseases, including eczema. However, as time went on it became clear that when they were taken regularly over a long period of time, oral steroids could have potentially serious side effects.

The main problem is that when oral steroids are taken over long periods, the adrenal glands shut down their own natural production of cortisol, with the result that the body is less able to deal effectively with injury or to fight off serious illness. Long-term oral steroids also have the effect of weakening the bones, consequently increasing the risk of osteoporosis in adults and stunted growth in children.

For this reason, strong oral steroids are only ever used to control cases of extremely severe atopic eczema, and even then only for as short a time as possible. In the rare instances where it is necessary to prescribe oral steroids, the doctor will keep a careful watch on the patient in order to minimize the undesirable side effects.

Topical steroids

Topical steroids in the form of creams, ointments, lotions or gels are a different matter entirely and have a very definite place in treating eczema. They come in various strengths or potencies: mild, moderate, strong and very strong, sometimes known by doctors as categories 1, 2, 3 and 4. The moderate, strong and very strong versions can be diluted to modify their potency, giving doctors a wide range of treatments to try.

The mild and moderate potencies (categories 1 and 2) that are most often used are quite safe, provided you follow a few common-sense precautions (see 'safe steroid use', page 67). In fact, the mildest preparations containing only 1 per cent hydrocortisone are available over the counter in the pharmacy and can be used without medical supervision.

Stronger topical steroids do have side effects including thin, transparent fragile skin which is prone to bruising, loss of skin elasticity and stretch marks, so they will only be prescribed to adults for a short period during flare-ups on areas of thick skin.

Topical steroids for adults and children The stronger potencies which your doctor may prescribe during a flare-up of eczema will be carefully tailored to you as an individual, taking into account your age, the extent of your eczema, its severity and any other medications you may be taking. The chart below shows a typical schedule for children and adults.

TOPICAL STEROID TREATMENT

	Adults	Children
Routine treatment	Moderate to strong (diluted) for the body. Mild to moderate for the face.	Mild to moderate for the body. Mild for the face.
Severe attacks	Strong for the body. Moderate for the face. Very strong for thick skin.	Diluted strong for the body. Moderate for the face.

Antibiotics and antiseptics

We all have germs living quite naturally on our skin. In normal circumstances they remain in balance and do no harm. However, because the skin is damaged in eczema sufferers, they may have more bacteria than usual on the skin surface. If these multiply, they can cause infection and this in turn may trigger a flare-up of eczema.

The most common culprit is a bacterium known as *Staphylococcus aureus*. Another culprit is Group A *Streptococcus*, a bacterium that also causes sore throats and tonsillitis. Signs of infection include worsening eczema symptoms with weeping and crusting, possibly combined with swollen glands and general feelings of illness. In the case of Group A streptococcal infection, a telltale sign of infection is a sore throat. The doctor may prescribe one of a number of antibiotics, and it is vital to complete the course, even though symptoms may disappear after a few days, in order to prevent resistance developing.

Attention to hygiene and skin care can help control bacteria on the skin. But if the infection doesn't clear up or you develop recurrent infections, the doctor may suggest you use an antiseptic solution in the bath or in the form of a wet compress. This can be especially useful where weeping is troublesome. The main drawbacks are that strong antiseptics can irritate already sensitive skin and can also be absorbed into the bloodstream.

Anti-histamines

Anti-histamines are drugs that block the effects of histamine, a chemical released as part of the body's allergic reaction. They

DRUG SIDE EFFECTS AND ALLERGIC REACTIONS

All drugs have beneficial effects and side effects. The term side effect is used to describe the body's reaction to a drug or other medication which is in addition to its therapeutic effect. Many of the drugs used in the treatment of eczema, including corticosteroids, can have side effects. Some of these may be serious and for this reason the doctor will always weigh the risks carefully against the benefits when prescribing any medication.

One possible side effect is an allergic reaction to the drug. This is one of the main problems with the use of topical anti-histamine drugs. The development of an allergic reaction to a topical anti-histamine may be especially problematic because this family of drugs is widely prescribed for many other conditions including asthma, hay fever, rhinitis and emotional problems such as anxiety. For this reason, most dermatologists avoid prescribing topical anti-histamines altogether for children with eczema. If you are worried about the possible side effects of your medication, contact your doctor.

are available as pills, capsules and syrups to be taken by mouth, and also as ointments, creams and lotions which can be applied directly to the skin.

Until fairly recently anti-histamines were frequently recommended for eczema as a way of reducing itching and thus combating the itch-scratch cycle. This was because it was thought that histamine was the main cause of itching. However, it has now become clear that the main advantage of anti-histamines is that some types cause drowsiness and it is this rather than any direct effect on itchiness that is responsible for the relief they provide. For this reason, topical anti-histamines are less likely to be prescribed, and many doctors prefer to prescribe older types of oral anti-histamine which have a more pronounced sedative effect.

Anti-histamines can be especially useful for children who have problems going to sleep or who wake during the night because of itching. However, the drugs have the opposite effect in a few children, making them hyperactive and even less able to sleep. Also, if used regularly, they may become less effective over time. For this reason, many experts recommend using them only on nights when the child is having great problems sleeping because of itching, or during acute flare-ups.

Bandages and wraps

A whole range of bandages and wraps are available which can be used to protect the skin, reduce inflammation and ease soreness and itching. In particular, so-called wet wrap dressings are growing in popularity for the treatment of severe eczema in babies and children. They have proved extremely effective in quelling inflammation and the tormenting itching that prevents so many children with eczema – and their parents – from getting a decent night's sleep.

Wet wrapping

The child's body, arms or legs are encased in tubular cotton bandages that have been soaked in warm water and applied over a layer of emollient cream or a weak steroid preparation. A dry bandage is then put over the top to form a kind of body suit. The treatment is applied after bathing and is left on overnight. The layered design helps keep the skin cool, quells itching and prevents scratching while enhancing the absorption of steroids. Once you become accustomed to them, the dressings are easy to apply and the whole process can usually be completed in under a quarter of an hour.

The use of wet wraps has transformed life for many children with eczema. Because they are so comfortable and soothing they enable the child to get a good night's sleep, sometimes for the first time ever. Once a child's eczema has been brought under control, he or she will usually only need to have a wet wrap during flare-ups.

Other bandages and dressings

Sometimes the doctor may suggest that bandages are used dry to make mittens or protect the skin to prevent night-time scratching. The doctor may also recommend various medicated bandages impregnated with coal-tar (see page 74), calamine or other medications to help cool and heal eczematous skin. There are also dressings made of a self-adhesive clear film which can be used with topical steroids to treat small areas of persistent eczema.

Immunosuppressive drugs

Because eczema is a disease of the immune system, in severe cases that do not respond to other milder forms of treatment, the doctor may sometimes prescribe one of a powerful family of drugs known as immunosuppressants. As the name suggests, these are drugs that suppress the action of the immune system. Unfortunately, these drugs can cause severe and potentially dangerous side effects, such as an increased likelihood of infection, anaemia and kidney problems.

The most commonly prescribed immunosuppressant is a drug called cyclosporine, which was originally developed to prevent the body rejecting organ transplants. The drug can sometimes have a dramatic effect in severe eczema. However, great care is needed in prescribing it because it can cause kidney damage. If the doctor thinks you would benefit, you are likely to be prescribed cyclosporine for no longer than 8–12 weeks and regular kidney function tests will be carried out to ensure that it is not causing any damage.

Azathioprine is another immunosuppressant drug which is also used to help patients who have had heart and kidney transplants. It may be prescribed to hold severe and chronic atopic eczema in check. It works by suppressing the activity of white blood cells. If the doctor thinks you would benefit from azathioprine, you will need to have regular blood and liver function tests.

Tar preparations

Tars – sticky secretions derived from various materials including coal, shale and wood – were traditionally used to soothe inflamed, itchy skin, and before more modern medical treatments became available, coal tar was often an effective treatment for eczema. However, its messiness and smelliness, together with the fact that it can be irritating, have caused it to fall out of favour. Various kinds of dilute coal-tar preparations, some mixed with steroid ointments and creams, are now available and can be useful. Other tars, such as ichthammol (derived from shale containing fossilized fish), are sometimes used in medicated bandages.

Light therapy

If you are one of those people who notices that your eczema improves when you go on holiday to a country with a sunny climate, you may benefit from phototherapy or light therapy. It involves exposing the body to light waves, either on their own or usually in combination with a drug called psoralen, which magnifies the effects of UVA radiation. Psoralen, which is derived from plants, can be given by mouth, applied to the skin as a lotion or dissolved in a bath. The treatment is used for mild to moderate eczema in children over 12 and adults. Because of possible side effects, including skin ageing and cancer, exposure to light waves is built up extremely slowly and kept to a minimum, as it should be with sunbathing. More recently, intensive types of phototherapy have been developed using special high-intensity lamps that emit different light wavelengths.

When hospital is necessary

Very occasionally, when treatments have not worked, an eczema sufferer may benefit from admission to hospital. A few days to a week in hospital can have a dramatic effect in clearing up a recalcitrant attack of eczema. Hospitalization enables an intensive treatment regimen that is not easy to maintain at home, and provides a break from common allergens such as house dust and animals, as well as a respite from the stresses and strains of everyday life.

Making the most of your doctor

You will control your eczema most effectively if you and your doctor can work in partnership. When you arrange a visit to the doctor's surgery, make sure you go armed with as much information about your eczema as possible (this is where your trigger diary can help). Be prepared to describe the course of your eczema: how often attacks occur, how long they last and whether they have changed over the course of time, together with details about how your life is affected when your eczema is active.

Make a note of any treatments you have tried, including over-the-counter remedies, prescribed medicines and complementary therapies, and whether they worked or not. This will help the doctor to decide on the most effective treatment regimen for you. Make a list of any questions you have about eczema or the drugs that may be prescribed to treat it.

5 Complementary treatments

Like any long-term condition, eczema can be extremely demoralizing. It is easy to begin to feel as if your life is ruled by your condition and by the medical treatments you have to use. You can soon begin to view yourself in rather negative terms as a 'patient' – someone who is unwell and helpless – with no control over your life.

Complementary therapies such as herbalism, homeopathy and hypnotherapy, with their emphasis on treating you as a whole person and helping the body to heal itself, can help you to feel much more positive and in control.

Although no complementary treatment has been proved to 'cure' eczema, the therapies can help to alleviate symptoms and make you feel better by helping you to feel less stressed. Until relatively recently, many orthodox doctors dismissed complementary therapies. However, this is now changing, partly as a result of increased consumer demand for a wider range of effective treatments.

Using complementary therapies

In the UK, eight out of ten people have tried a complementary therapy of some sort and three-quarters of those felt that they had benefited. Research has shown that complementary therapies can be extremely effective in conditions such as eczema which are often made worse by stress. Many orthodox dermatologists are also taking a keen interest in the use of Chinese herbs, which have been shown to be extremely effective as a treatment for some adults and children whose eczema is difficult to control with orthodox treatments.

If you do decide to give complementary therapies a try, it is important to be aware that they are complementary, that is they are intended to be used alongside conventional medicine or medication, and not to replace it. You should never stop using any medication you have been prescribed without first discussing it with your orthodox doctor.

Another important point to remember is that, just as with orthodox treatment, there is no one therapy that works for everyone. Just because Chinese herbal treatment has helped some people with eczema does not mean that it will work for you. Each one of us is different and our bodies respond differently to different regimens, and this applies to conventional medical treatment too. So be patient and be prepared for some trial and error in finding the therapy or therapies that work best for you. It can sometimes take quite a while before you experience any improvement.

On the other hand, you should not persist with a treatment that seems to be having no therapeutic effect. You should always ask the complementary practitioner how long you should expect to wait before experiencing an improvement.

Finding a therapist

As complementary therapies become more widely accepted and used, many of the complementary therapy organizations are becoming more tightly regulated. However, as yet there is no one governing body for complementary therapists as there is for orthodox medical practitioners, so it is very much your responsibility to find a reputable practitioner.

Your local phone directory can provide you with a list of complementary therapy organizations and registered practitioners. However, their standards do vary. Therefore, don't be afraid to ask for details of what sort of training and qualifications their members have to undergo and whether this is on a full-time or part-time basis. Check the premises to make sure that they are clean and well-run: you should expect the same standards of hygiene and professionalism as from an orthodox doctor.

Once you have found a practitioner in your area, you need to ask a few pertinent questions. These include:

❑ What qualifications do they have?
❑ How did they acquire them?
❑ How long have they been practising?
❑ How long is treatment likely to take?
❑ How much will treatment cost?

The relationship between you and your practitioner is an important part of your treatment, so it is vital to find someone whom you feel you can trust. Beware of anyone who promises you a miracle cure or anyone you feel uncomfortable with for whatever reason.

The first appointment

One of the features of most forms of complementary medicine is that the practitioner will look at you as a whole person and not just treat your symptoms. For this reason, a first appointment with a complementary practitioner tends to last much longer than the average doctor's appointment – usually an hour or more. The practitioner will take a detailed medical history and will ask you about your symptoms, what treatments you have had and why you are seeking treatment. He or she will also need details of your lifestyle, your diet, your work, your exercise habits, your stress levels and so on, in order to establish a broader picture of your eczema within the context of you and your life. You should also expect to answer questions about your overall health and details of your family medical history, so it is a good idea to go armed with this information at the outset.

Depending on the type of therapy you are seeking, there may then follow a physical examination. The therapist will usually want to see your rash and establish its nature – whether it is dry or wet, and so on. He or she may also want to take your pulse (or pulses in the case of Chinese practitioners), listen to your heart and perform blood or urine tests.

Which therapy to choose

There are many potentially useful complementary treatments for eczema. The following is a brief selection of the ones that have been found to be useful for some people. However, they are not the only therapies that may help. If you like the idea of trying a particular therapy, try and find out as much about it beforehand and ask other people with eczema if they have found it helpful. Eczema organizations will usually be willing to advise on treatments their members have found effective.

Acupuncture

Acupuncture, like Chinese herbal treatment, is part of a much wider tradition of Oriental healing going back some 5,000 years, which also includes acupressure, moxibustion (when smouldering herbs are applied near acupuncture points), herbs, massage, diet and exercises such as t'ai chi. Collectively these different treatments are known as traditional Chinese medicine (TCM). With the growing interest in complementary medical treatment nowadays, many people are turning to TCM for help with allergies like eczema, asthma and hayfever.

Acupuncture involves the insertion of fine needles into the skin at points known as acupoints. These lie along invisible lines called meridians, down which the body's life force, 'qi' or 'chi', is said to flow.

The concept of chi is part of an extremely complex system of philosophy of the Dao, or 'the path of life'. However, put simply, according to Chinese philosophy, it is the blockage or stagnation of chi that causes disease. The aim of acupuncture is to stimulate the flow of chi, calm overactive chi and remove any blockages, thus helping the body to heal itself.

The most important idea in Chinese philosophy is that of harmony and balance. According to the Chinese view, we are all governed by the interplay of two opposing forces known as 'yin' and 'yang'. Although these are not readily understood in Western terms, broadly speaking yin is the female force and is associated with cold, darkness, damp and internal factors, while yang is the male force associated with warmth, light, heat and external factors. According to Chinese thinking, when these two forces are in balance our bodies are healthy. However, if they become unbalanced, the result is disease.

Chinese philosophy also involves an understanding of what are known as the five elements – wood, fire, earth, metal and water. Each of these is linked to a season, an organ, a taste, colour, smell, emotion or body part. Again, the system is based on the idea that our lives and our bodies are in a process of constant change, a never-ending cycle which is part of the balance of nature. For anyone brought up in the Western medical tradition, with its emphasis on scientific thinking, this can sound a little doubtful. However, although the concepts are strange, they are useful as a way of understanding that physical disease can affect us on all sorts of levels. For example, an attack of eczema can be triggered by the emotions or affected by our environment, the climate, the seasons, diet and exercise.

According to acupuncture theory, the skin condition eczema is linked to exposure to damp, heat and wind. If you think about it, this is not so different from the ancient Greek description of 'boiling over'.

An acupuncture consultation

During the first consultation, the practitioner will employ his or her five senses to reach a diagnosis: looking, asking, listening, smelling and touching. He or she will ask you details about your life and lifestyle, will look at your appearance and posture, the colour of your face, the brightness of your eyes and the appearance of your tongue (a healthy tongue is light red with a moist, thin, whitish coating). He or she will listen to your breathing, note the tone of your voice and how you cough, and will take your pulses. There are three pulse points on each wrist, according to acupuncture theory, and 28 different qualities of pulse that help guide the practitioner to the source of your disease. The practitioner will then devise a course of treatment specifically designed to restore your chi and to bring your body back into balance. As well as the actual acupuncture treatment, this may involve advice on your diet, lifestyle and the use of Chinese herbs (see pages 85–7).

Although many people dislike the idea of having needles inserted, acupuncture treatment is rarely painful. The application of the needles may be felt as a pinprick followed by numbness or tingling and some people may feel a slight ache. The acupuncturist will manipulate the needles to stimulate or calm the point being treated. This can take anything from minutes to hours.

After treatment, people report feeling a number of different sensations. Some people feel extremely tired, others say they are full of energy. It is common to experience a temporary worsening of symptoms before there is an improvement but you would normally expect to start feeling better after three or four treatments. Discuss it with your practitioner and ask when he or she would expect your skin symptoms to clear up. However if you don't start to see an improvement after this amount of time, it could well be that acupuncture treatment is not for you. Don't forget to inform your orthodox medical practitioner that you are having acupuncture treatment.

Herbal treatments

Herbs have been used throughout the ages all over the world to treat and cure illness. In fact, many conventional pharmaceutical drugs are based on the active ingredients found in herbs, and even today 80 per cent of the world's population relies on herbal remedies for the treatment of illness and disease. Aspirin, for example, originally derives from the bark of the white willow, which has been known for centuries for its anti-inflammatory properties, while the active ingredient in the humble foxglove is digitalis, a heartbeat regulator which is the basis of the medical drug dixogin.

Herbalists believe that disease is caused by the body trying to cure itself. Herbal remedies therefore are prescribed to

SAFETY NOTE

Herbal remedies have stood the test of time and are often much safer than conventional pharmaceutical drugs. However, this does not mean you should assume they are completely safe. Herbal treatments have a pharmacological action, that is they change your body chemistry just like conventional drugs, and can be toxic if taken in large doses or mixed with other drugs or even other complementary treatments. For this reason, it is important to tell your doctor about your herbal remedies, and your herbalist about any conventional medication you are taking. To be on the safe side, never take herbs during pregnancy or give herbal remedies to a baby or child without the advice of a qualified medical herbalist.

support the immune system as it fights off illness as well as to combat the symptoms of disease. This can be especially important in conditions such as eczema which arise from an overreactive immune system.

Chinese herbal treatment

Chinese herbalism, like acupuncture, is part of traditional Chinese medicine. It involves using mixtures of herbs made up into teas or decoctions to treat and prevent disease. In the past few years there has been a tremendous amount of interest in the use of Chinese herbs for eczema, following the remarkable success of two medical trials which showed that children and adults with difficult-to-treat eczema experienced a 60 per cent improvement in their symptoms following treatment with Chinese herbs.

Because of the way in which orthodox scientific trials are conducted, how the herbs were used was somewhat different to the way they are normally used in traditional Chinese medicine (TCM). In TCM, patients are diagnosed individually and the herbs prescribed are tailored to the particular person rather than the illness. By contrast, in controlled scientific studies, it is vital for the patients treated to be as alike as possible and for the treatment to be exactly the same, so as to assess objectively the effects of treatment on the symptoms. In the hospital trials described above, therefore, patients were chosen with the same symptoms and the herbal mixture was a standard mixture of ten herbs ground up and packed into special tea bags.

Research is currently under way to try to identify potentially active ingredients in the herbs used, again a rather different approach to the traditional Chinese way. Like acupuncture, Chinese herbs work to restore the flow of chi and the balance of yin and yang.

In the Chinese philosophy of yin and yang, acupuncture is yang because it moves from the outside in, while herbs are considered to be yin because they move from the inside out. Treatment for eczema consists of rebalancing heat and damp in the body and repairing the stomach, lung and kidney functions, which are considered to be disturbed according to Chinese thinking.

Some orthodox doctors are very excited by Chinese herbs, especially as they seem to be useful in cases of eczema that have proved impossible to control by any other means. In his book *Eczema in childhood: the facts*, Paediatric dermatologist Dr David Atherton, who is based at the world-famous Great Ormond Street Hospital for Sick Children in London, hailed Chinese herbs as 'the first effective new treatment for atopic eczema since topical steroids were introduced'.

In the United Kingdom Chinese herbal treatment used to be available on the National Health Service. However, this is no longer the case. If you would like to try Chinese herbal treatment it is a good idea to discuss it thoroughly with your doctor or dermatologist at the hospital. This is an important precaution in case the treatment may interact with any orthodox treatments you have been prescribed. Your doctor may want to keep an eye on your liver function during treatment to avoid any adverse effects.

The Chinese approach places an emphasis on prescribing herbs for you as an individual. If you decide to take this route, it is very important to seek the help of a qualified Chinese herbal practitioner who is registered with the Register of Chinese Herbal Medicine. Chinese herbs are prescribed to take into account the individual's whole symptom picture and many herbs are not safe for unsupervised use. That is why it is important to have a prescription made up especially for you and never to take a remedy that has been prescribed for someone else. Practitioners of Chinese herbal medicine are trained to diagnose and treat people with herbal remedies. The herbal pharmacists, who often have shops on the high street, are qualified to dispense herbs but are not registered to practise herbal medicine. Although some Chinese practitioners use the title Doctor, legally this only applies to medical doctors. There have been (admittedly fairly rare) reports of problems with allergic reactions to the herbs which can affect the liver. Consequently, it is important that you have regular blood checks to ensure that your bone marrow, kidneys and liver are not being damaged by the treatment in any way. If you feel unwell, nauseous or develop diarrhoea or flu-like symptoms while taking Chinese herbs, stop taking them straight away and contact your practitioner.

Because of the danger of liver problems, Chinese herbs should never be used by anyone who has had liver problems such as jaundice or hepatitis, or by children who are taking any other medication.

Medical herbalism (Western herbalism)

Like Chinese herbal treatment, medical herbalism or Western herbalism involves using plants and herbs (usually those that grow in Western countries) to maintain health and keep the body in balance. The aim of treatment is to support the body

USING HERBAL REMEDIES

Herbal remedies come in many different forms. They can be taken internally in the form of infusions (teas made from flowers and leaves), decoctions (teas made from the woody parts of plants such as the bark or roots), as tablets or capsules or in tinctures (made by soaking herbs in alcohol). Alternatively, they can be applied externally as compresses or poultices, in creams and ointments or in herbal baths.

during illness and to stimulate the body's own healing energy which may have been weakened by factors such as stress, lack of exercise, poor nutrition and external environmental factors such as pollution.

The main difference between herbal medicine and orthodox medicine is that, whereas in pharmaceutical drugs one or more active ingredients are isolated, herbalists believe that using the whole herb is more beneficial. Many of the other ingredients a plant contains have a buffering effect which helps to prevent unwelcome side effects. In addition, the chemical complexity of herbs means that they can often achieve more than a drug with just one active ingredient. Some herbs are known as adaptogens, meaning that they act to rebalance the body, depending on what the body needs.

A herbal consultation

As with many kinds of complementary medicine, the typical consultation with a medical herbalist usually lasts much longer than a consultation with a conventional doctor. The herbalist will take details of your symptoms, your lifestyle, your personality and your family medical history and will also note details such as your appearance, the condition of your hair and skin, the way you move and so on. The idea is to look for underlying causes of your disease rather than just treating the symptoms. Thus in the case of eczema, the herbalist may well treat the underlying immune problem that is causing your rash (see 'herbs for eczema', below) rather than the rash itself. Very often you will be prescribed something to alleviate your skin symptoms in the meantime. Burdock, elder flowers, chickweed, marigold, witch hazel and yellow dock may be prescribed as compresses to alleviate inflammation and heal pustules.

The remedies prescribed will be tailored to you, not to your symptoms, which is why it is better to see a medical herbalist rather than buying an off-the-shelf product for treating eczema. The herbalist may also advise you on diet and food intolerance, and on avoiding irritants. As with other complementary treatments, you may feel worse rather than better at first. This is seen as the body ridding itself of toxins and beginning the process of healing.

HERBS FOR ECZEMA

To relieve pain and itching	To reduce inflammation	To boost the immune system
Chamomile	Chamomile	Echinacea
Calendula	Burdock	Nettles
	Calendula	Yarrow
	Red clover	

Homeopathy

Homeopathy is a system of medicine based on the philosophy of like treating like – substances that cause symptoms in someone who is well are used in homeopathic remedies to cure the same symptoms in someone who is unwell. The idea is that the remedy stimulates the body's own self-healing mechanisms. According to homeopathic thinking, symptoms are an expression of the body's attempt to heal itself. Homeopathic remedies are designed to stimulate the body's healing mechanism in a similar fashion to the way vaccines are given in conventional medicine.

The substances used in homeopathic remedies are derived from plants, minerals and animal sources. They are used in minute amounts which are not detectable by conventional chemical analysis. The remedies are made by preparing a strained solution of the main ingredient, known as the mother tincture. This is repeatedly strained and diluted, and shaken or 'succussed', before being made into tablets, pills, granules or powder – homeopathic remedies are usually taken in the form of small lactose tablets. The strength of the remedy or its potency depends on the number of times it has been diluted but, contrary to what you might imagine, the more times a remedy has been diluted, the higher its potency. A remedy of the sixth potency (written as 6c), the lowest potency, which is available for self-treatment from health food shops and pharmacies, has been diluted six times in a ratio of 1 drop of the mother tincture to 99 drops of an alcohol and water mix.

By and large, there are two main types of remedies – constitutional remedies which are prescribed for you as a person, and more specific remedies designed to treat symptoms which can be used at home for self-treatment. Because eczema is such a complex illness, it is preferable to see a homeopath and be prescribed a constitutional remedy rather than trying self-treatment. Both over-the-counter items and homeopathic prescriptions are available from a homeopathic dispensary.

Orthodox doctors cannot offer scientific explanation for how homeopathy might work because the active ingredients are present in such small quantities that they cannot possibly have a pharmacological effect. Homeopaths argue that it is the remedy's vital energy or 'vibrational pattern' rather than its particular ingredients that stimulates healing.

One of the most important principles of homeopathy is whole-person prescribing. Treatment is aimed at you as a person with a particular set of symptoms rather than at the symptoms, as it is in conventional medicine. This means that a homeopath will not treat eczema; he will treat someone with eczematous symptoms. While an orthodox doctor will broadly prescribe the same treatments for everyone with eczema, the homeopath might well prescribe a different remedy depending on how eczema affects you as a person.

In fact, homeopathy has been found to be very effective in treating allergies and skin complaints. In two trials, patients with skin conditions characteristic of the homeopathic remedy sulphur, with symptoms such as diarrhoea, thirst, itching and heat-sensitivity, were treated with either sulphur or a dummy remedy. Around half of those treated responded to the homeopathic treatment, but none of those treated with the dummy remedy showed a response. At the end of the trials, 58 per cent of those treated experienced a permanent improvement in their symptoms.

A homeopathic consultation

In the UK, some homeopaths are orthodox doctors who have trained in homeopathy. Others are lay practitioners who have completed a minimum three-year homeopathy course. The practitioner will take details of your history and ask you lots of questions both about your eczema and about you. The idea is to get as full a picture as possible which can then be matched to a remedy. Some of the questions may seem rather unusual compared to an orthodox medical consultation, and might include what sort of weather you prefer, whether your symptoms are worse for heat or cold and what sort of food you like.

Taking a homeopathic remedy is quite different from a conventional treatment. The remedy must be taken in a 'clean' mouth, that is, you should not have had a cup of coffee or tea, smoked a cigarette or even cleaned your teeth before taking it. Remedies of the lowest 6c potency may well be prescribed for use every two hours until you begin to feel better, and thereafter three times a day. More potent remedies may well be prescribed as a single pill to be taken once a day for three days. Very often there will be a worsening of symptoms before you

HOMEOPATHIC REMEDIES FOR ECZEMA

Remedy	Symptoms
Graphites	Moist rash with yellowish discharge; dry, cracked or rough skin especially behind ears and on hands. Inherited.
Petroleum	Moist eczema with rough, broken skin. Brought on by stress or allergy.
Sulphur	Dry, rough, red itchy rash. Brought on by allergy or inherited tendency.

begin to feel better. This is regarded as a good sign because it is said to 'prove' the remedy. Sometimes the homeopath may then prescribe further remedies as the old symptoms disappear and new ones come to the surface.

Hypnosis

Hypnosis or hypnotherapy is especially useful in stress-related conditions such as eczema, and can also be useful in helping to combat eczematous symptoms such as heat and itching. When used therapeutically – rather than for entertainment – hypnosis is a form of psychotherapy that is used to access a person's subconscious mind. Hypnosis can be employed to tackle stress by helping people change their thoughts and behaviour patterns, in order to enable them to deal more effectively with stressful events in their lives.

The hypnotherapist uses a number of simple relaxation techniques to induce a hypnotic trance, a level of consciousness that is somewhere between wakefulness and sleeping, akin to the state the brain is in during meditation. In this state, barriers are broken down making the mind more responsive. Different therapists work in different ways. The type of hypnosis many people are most familiar with, in which the therapist gives the client direct suggestions or commands to do something, is known as command hypnotherapy. Although this type of hypnotherapy has its uses, for example for calming exam nerves or getting rid of bad habits such as smoking, many hypnotherapists prefer to work at a more subtle level, making use of techniques such as deep relaxation and visualization, in which you are encouraged to use the power of your imagination to control symptoms and aid healing. For example, you may be encouraged to visualize healthy skin cells growing in number and pushing out the unhealthy skin cells. Alternatively, you may be asked to imagine yourself rolling in the snow to cool and soothe a hot, red, itchy rash.

A hypnotherapy consultation

A first consultation will usually last for 1–1½ hours, with subsequent sessions taking just under an hour. The hypnotherapist will want to know about your symptoms, what has caused you to come for hypnotherapy and what you hope to get out of it. A great deal of time is usually devoted to building up a sense of trust between the therapist and the client. It is especially important to seek the help of a qualified medical hypnotherapist. Do not be afraid to ask questions and if you feel at all uncomfortable with the therapist, for whatever reason, there is no need for you to go ahead with treatment.

The therapist may hypnotize you during the first session but often this is not done until the second session. It involves helping you to attain a deep relaxation. Bear in mind that even while you are in a trance, you are in control and the therapist cannot make you do anything you do not want to do. The therapist may well teach you how to hypnotize yourself and may give you a tape to take home to help you go into a trance, for use when you need help to relax and sleep, or to calm itching. Hypnotherapy is not suitable for children under seven.

Naturopathy

Naturopathy is an approach towards healing that makes use of natural resources, such as the food we eat, the water we drink or bathe in and the air we breathe, to help the body heal itself. Naturopaths regard disease as a natural phenomenon brought out by the body getting out of balance through poor diet, lack of exercise, harmful emotions, the accumulation of toxins, inherited factors and an unhealthy environment. They also believe that the body possesses a vital force that enables it to heal itself.

The aim of treatment is to support the body as it heals itself. The symptoms of disease are signs that the body is trying to heal itself, and they should therefore be encouraged and not suppressed. The occasional cold, for example, is seen as a healthy way for the body to eliminate toxins and strengthen the immune system. Intriguingly, orthodox medicine may be coming round to this idea. Research shows that children who do not have many colds and minor infections in early life are more at risk of developing eczema.

Diet is one of the most important tools in naturopathy and there is an emphasis on eating whole, organic foods and plenty of fruit and vegetables – just the sort of diet that is increasingly being recommended for good health. Where allergies and intolerances are involved, as they may be in eczema, elimination diets can be an important part of treatment. You can read more about dietary strategies in Chapter 6, pages 99–120.

Other treatment tactics may include fasting (to rest the digestive system and help rid the body of toxins), hydrotherapy (the use of water in the form of compresses, cold or hot baths, saunas and so on), massage, osteopathy and psychotherapy. Some naturopaths are also trained in other complementary therapies, such as homeopathy or herbalism, and may use these where appropriate.

Reflexology and yoga

Physical therapies, like reflexology and yoga, are both useful in calming the mind and relaxing the body which, given that eczema often gets worse under stress, can be tremendously helpful in keeping the condition under control. Ancient Indian statues show that yoga was practised in northern India some 4,000 years ago. The principles of hatha yoga (which concentrates on the physical) were laid down in the eighth century by the Indian teacher Pantajali and in essence remain the same today.

Reflexology too has its origins in the ancient world – in this case, in the civilizations of Egypt, India, China, Africa and the American Indians. However it did not make any impact in the West until early in the 20th century when the US physician Dr William Fitzgerald became interested in what he called 'zone therapy'. The practice of this therapy was subsequently taken up by Dr Joe Riley and physiotherapist Eunice Ingham who coined the term reflexology.

Reflexology

Reflexology, or zone therapy, involves applying pressure to points in the feet and hands in order to stimulate the body's own healing mechanisms. Reflexologists believe that the different parts of the body are mirrored on the feet and hands, and that by stimulating points corresponding to that organ, healing can occur.

Zone therapy is said to be effective in lifting tension and stress, reducing inflammation and helping the body to rid itself of toxins. All these things mean that it is a useful therapy to try if you have eczema.

Yoga

Yoga is a gentle movement system which helps to bring body and mind into harmony through a series of asanas, or postures. There are many different types of yoga. However, the one most popular in the West is hatha yoga which involves learning different methods of breathing (pranayama), designed to encourage relaxation and concentration, the practice of asanas (postures) and dhyana, or meditation. The breathing helps to make full use of the lungs and encourages the body to expel toxins, while practising the asanas uses all the body's muscles to help attain strength and flexibility and release tension. Meditation helps to relax the mind, so it can be especially useful in controlling stress, which is often a trigger for eczema.

A yoga session would typically include 10 minutes of relaxation and breath control, followed by 15–20 minutes warm-up, 25 minutes of postures and 20 minutes more of relaxation. The class may end with 5–10 minutes of reflection and/or chanting. With its mind-body approach, yoga can bring real benefits to eczema sufferers, both physical and mental.

Therapy safety

❑ Ask people you know with eczema if they know of any local complementary therapists. Always ask how satisfied they were with treatment. Self-help groups also have guidelines. Alternatively, your doctor, pharmacist or health visitor may know of qualified practitioners in your area.

❑ Get in touch with the therapy's professional organization who should be able to tell you the names of practitioners in your area. They should also supply you with details of training and their code of professional practice.

❑ When you first contact a practitioner, ask him or her how many treatments they anticipate you will need, how much each session will cost and when you can expect to experience an improvement. In many of these therapies, there is a temporary worsening of symptoms initially. This 'healing crisis' is usually regarded as a positive sign that the body is beginning to heal itself. However, symptoms should not continue to get worse.

❑ Recognize that there is no 'cure' for eczema and beware of any practitioner who offers you the promise of a miracle treatment.

❑ Always tell both your orthodox doctor and your complementary practitioner of any treatment you are prescribed as sometimes there are adverse reactions between, say, herbs and conventional drugs.

❑ Never stop taking your orthodox medical treatment without getting your doctor's permission.

6 Food and eczema

Much controversy and argument surrounds the idea that food may play a role in triggering eczema. Some people are convinced that certain foods make their skin worse, while avoiding them makes it better.

Until fairly recently, many orthodox doctors dismissed the idea that food had a significant role to play in eczema, except for the small percentage of young children who are allergic to cows' milk. However, in recent years this view has changed. A great deal more has come to be understood about the ways in which a sensitivity to food can spark off a number of adverse reactions in the body.

It is now generally acknowledged that some 10–25 per cent of people are affected by food sensitivity and it is becoming much more widely accepted that such sensitivity may play a part in some cases of eczema. In fact, according to current estimates, food sensitivity is now thought to be a factor in almost one-third of cases of children with atopic eczema.

A word of caution

Dietary measures alone are unlikely to have an effect on any but the mildest eczema. However, they can make an effective weapon in the armoury against eczema and that can only be a good thing. But because eczema is a multi-factorial disease (that is, it is caused by a combination of different factors), there is no single treatment that works for everyone. As we have seen, many people with eczema are helped by emollient therapy, combined with avoiding environmental irritants. Many need medical treatment, at least part of the time, some may find help in complementary therapies, while others may benefit by avoiding certain foods or from taking nutritional supplements. However, in all but the mildest cases, treatment is likely to be complex. Don't expect miracles, and if you do decide to go the dietary route, be sure to seek help from a qualified dietitian, nutritionist or a doctor who specializes in nutrition and allergy. Babies and children, in particular, should never be put on a severely restricted diet without seeking medical advice.

Staying healthy

One of the simplest things you can do to stay healthy and help your body to heal itself is to eat a nutritious diet. Such a diet will help boost the health of your immune system and will also provide you with the energy you need to help you cope with the stress of your condition. Until recently, most of the emphasis in dietary advice for allergies has been on cutting out certain foods. In the past few years, a great deal of excitement has been generated by the discovery that certain nutrients actively help to fight disease. There are literally hundreds of these compounds, known as phyto-chemicals (from the Greek *phyto* meaning plant), present in common foods. This is a tremendous step forward because it means to stay healthy the emphasis is less on what you can't eat and instead is on what you can eat.

The ability to stay healthy is literally on your plate. Some of the nutrients that have been found to be helpful in relieving eczema are outlined on pages 120, but it is likely that more will be discovered as further research is conducted.

Food and your skin

As we have seen, the skin is the body's largest organ, so it is not really surprising to learn that a nutritious diet is crucial to its health. Shortages of particular vitamins, minerals and trace elements can show up in the skin – whether or not you have eczema. However, if you do have eczema it is especially important to pay attention to eating a healthy diet. In fact, if the eczema is mild, sometimes eating a more nutritious diet, combined with the self-help measures outlined in previous chapters, can improve your skin health without the need for any other dietary measures. If you have severe eczema, you will usually need to combine a sensible eating regime (and possibly a special diet) with medical treatment.

So what should you eat to maintain a healthy skin? The key is to eat a well-balanced diet. Rather than setting rigid rules about what you should and shouldn't eat, nutritionists and dietitians today concentrate on maintaining a healthy balance. To achieve this they suggest that you visualize your daily food intake as a plate of different foods.

The largest portion on your plate should be unrefined carbohydrates: starchy foods such as wholemeal bread, pasta, brown rice, couscous and starchy fruits and vegetables, for instance potatoes, squash, yams, plantains and bananas. These are the foods you need for sustained energy levels – of vital importance for all of us but especially for anyone living with a chronic condition such as eczema, which can be very draining.

The next biggest portion on your plate should be fruits and vegetables. You should select a good mixture of green leafy varieties such as cabbage, spinach, broccoli and lettuce, together with red, yellow and green varieties such as peppers, carrots, tomatoes, courgettes and so on. Fruits and vegetables are an important source of nutrients known as antioxidants, which are especially important for healthy skin. These are nutrients that act within the body's cells to combat the damage caused by rogue molecules known as free-radicals, which are now thought to be involved in a whole host of diseases and in ageing. The main antioxidants are vitamin A (or beta-carotene, which is changed in the body into vitamin A), vitamin C and vitamin E – known as the ACE vitamins – together with the trace mineral selenium. Another group of nutrients in fruits and vegetables, called quercetins, is said to stabilize cell membranes and thus block the allergic response.

The next portion on your plate should be protein foods. You need these to repair and maintain your body's tissues, and also to help strengthen your immune system. Protein is found in meat, poultry, game, fish, eggs, dairy products, beans, peas, nuts and seeds. An important nutrient for the skin, which is found in protein foods such as oysters, clams, eggs, hazelnuts, Brazil nuts and pumpkin seeds, is the mineral zinc. Zinc is vital for healing, and a shortage has been linked to a variety of skin problems including eczema.

Last of all, making up the smallest portion, your diet should include some fats, oils and, if you want, a very small amount of sugary foods. The fats that are especially important in eczema are two groups of fatty acids known as omega-6 and omega-3. These are found in nuts and seeds and their oils (especially cold pressed), and in oily fish such as sardines, herrings, salmon and tuna. A shortage of these essential fatty acids is associated with the development of dry skin, the very last thing you want if you are prone to eczema. They are

---

GENERAL DIET FOR A HEALTHY SKIN

○ Eat plenty of fresh fruit and vegetables, organic if at all possible.

○ Keep your intake of saturated fats (found in meat, full-fat cheeses and dairy foods) to a minimum.

○ Include essential fatty acids found in nuts, seeds, vegetable oils (such as olive oil) and oily fish.

○ Drink plenty of water and herbal teas.

○ Avoid too many caffeine-containing beverages such as coffee, tea, cocoa and cola-type drinks.

○ Consider cutting out histamine-containing foods such as ripened cheeses, red wine, salami and other cured sausages.

important because they are converted in the body into hormone-like substances called prostaglandins, which are involved in quelling inflammation.

This important process can be blocked by a diet that contains too many saturated fats (of the kind found in meat, butter and full-fat cheese) and fried foods, so at the same time as increasing your intake of omega-3 and omega-6 fatty acids, you should also be cutting down on animal fats and fatty foods such as pastries, biscuits and cakes.

It is worth mentioning two other substances that should be avoided if at all possible if you are prone to allergy and food sensitivity. The first is caffeine, found in tea, coffee, chocolate and cola-type drinks. Although caffeine is not generally directly involved in eczema, it can have the effect of irritating the gut lining and making it more permeable, which in turn can make you more likely to develop a food sensitivity. If you simply can't do without your cups of coffee or tea, try making them weaker than you normally would.

The other substance that you should be wary of is the chemical histamine, found in foods such as ripened cheeses, red wine and smoked and cured sausages, for example salami. Histamine is part of the chemical cascade involved in allergic reactions, so cutting out foods that contain histamine may be helpful in controlling your eczema.

Food sensitivity

In the past decade, scientists have come to understand a great deal more about the interaction between diet and eczema. The subject of food sensitivity is enormously complicated, but broadly speaking there are two potential reactions to food.

Immediate food hypersensitivity

The first reaction is a true allergic reaction, sometimes called immediate food hypersensitivity. This is a very specific response that happens almost immediately – usually within minutes and certainly no more than a couple of hours – after ingesting or even coming into contact with a particular food. In this type of reaction, the body wrongly identifies the food you have consumed as a foreign body and responds by releasing specific antibodies – in particular the allergy antibody IgE which, as we have already seen, is involved in the allergic response to fight off the potential invader.

Research suggests that many people who react to food have a leaky gut wall. The gut wall is designed to let through some molecules as part of the process of digestion, but sometimes it can become over-permeable as a result of stress, irritants such as coffee and alcohol and certain medications. When this happens, molecules of half-digested food enter the bloodstream triggering the release of chemicals such as histamine, which are responsible for symptoms like nettle rash (urticaria), swelling and redness. These may be accompanied by other symptoms such as wheezing, itchy eyes and sneezing.

The foods that trigger this response are often proteins – for example, wheat, milk and peanuts – and only a small amount of food is needed to set off a reaction. Sometimes even as little as handling a plate containing the food or kissing someone who has been eating the food can be enough to trigger an allergic reaction. True food hypersensitivity of this kind, especially to eggs and cows' milk, is most common in babies and small children and will normally disappear by the time the child is five.

Because food allergy involves a specific immune response, it is possible to test for it using various tests such as the RAST test (see page 110).

Delayed food hypersensitivity

The second type of reaction to food, variously called food intolerance, masked food allergy or delayed food hypersensitivity, is rather more complicated. In this type of reaction, symptoms develop some time after eating the food in question – usually 6–24 hours but sometimes longer – and effects can last for several hours or days.

There is much controversy about delayed food hypersensitivity and doctors still do not fully understand the underlying mechanism that triggers it. However, there are several key factors that are associated with the reaction which can help you determine whether it is this or immediate food hypersensitivity that is causing your symptoms.

First, the foods that trigger delayed hypersensitivity are usually everyday foods – often a mainstay of your diet. Unlike food allergy, where only a minute amount of a food can trigger a reaction, they also tend to be foods that you consume in large quantities. That is why in Europe, foods like wheat and milk are commonly implicated, whereas in countries such as China and India, people are more likely to be sensitive to rice. Usually people are sensitive to a fairly small number – between one and five foods – but sometimes people start off by being sensitive to a small range of foods but develop sensitivities to more and more foods as time goes on.

Secondly, symptoms often come and go. You may well be fine eating a particular food one day but on another day the same food item may cause a reaction. Very often the culprits are foods you have been eating for many years without any significant problems.

Thirdly, you may experience a variety of symptoms rather than one clear-cut reaction – itching, headaches, fatigue, fluid retention, irritability or depression, muscle and joint aches, low blood sugar (hypoglycaemia), flushes, sweats, diarrhoea, constipation, 'wind' and indigestion.

Curiously, people with delayed food hypersensitivity often crave the very foods and beverages to which they are intolerant. In fact, one of the key features of delayed food hypersensitivity is that when you stop consuming a food or drink to which you are intolerant, you often feel worse before you feel better. This is a result of withdrawal – a bit like quitting smoking or coming off an addictive drug.

Just to complicate matters further, if you are atopic (that is you have a tendency to allergies) and have a history of allergies such as hay fever, asthma, rhinitis and eczema, you are particularly at risk of both delayed food hypersensitivity and true food allergy.

Taking action

So what should you do if you think food is a factor in your eczema? What foods can you eat and what should you avoid?

It is worth making the point yet again that the approach taken will depend on whether you are an adult with eczema or the parent of a child with eczema. The severe exclusion diets sometimes used to treat severe adult eczema can be extremely unsafe for children and should never be undertaken without medical advice. In fact, many experts insist that food exclusion should only be tried when eczema is so bad that it is significantly disrupting the child's life. Children with mild eczema whose symptoms are controlled by self-help measures and the use of a mild steroid ointment or cream, they argue, rarely need to change their eating habits unless they are also experiencing other symptoms such as those outlined above.

Keeping a food diary

Because there is no single reliable test for food sensitivity, one of the most important factors in identifying potential triggers is your own observation. Keeping a food diary in which you note down everything consumed is a useful way of detecting whether there is any significant pattern of reaction to a particular food or foods. As well as noting down what is eaten, you should note any symptoms, such as a worsening of itching, redness or swelling, difficulty sleeping, headache, joint pains, digestive symptoms, fatigue and so on. Over a period of 4–6 weeks you may begin to see a pattern emerge.

Common offending foods

Experts in food sensitivity say that a mere seven foods are responsible for some 90 per cent of food-sensitive reactions. They are peanuts, shellfish, tree nuts (such as pecans and walnuts), eggs, milk, soya and wheat. In eczema, the most common culprits are cows' milk and eggs. However, white fish, yeast, fruits, caffeine and corn can also cause significant problems for many people. In fact, almost any food can trigger a reaction, which is why keeping a diary is so useful. It enables you to pinpoint possible culprits that affect you. The following foods are common culprits in food sensitivity.

- [ ] Wheat, rye, oats, corn
- [ ] Dairy products – milk, cheese and hens' eggs
- [ ] Beef
- [ ] Poultry
- [ ] White fish
- [ ] Shellfish
- [ ] Chocolate, tea, coffee
- [ ] Food additives
- [ ] Yeast
- [ ] Pork
- [ ] Peanuts
- [ ] Tree nuts e.g. hazelnuts, almonds, walnuts, pecans
- [ ] Soya beans
- [ ] Bananas
- [ ] Citrus fruits
- [ ] Alcohol

Testing for allergy

Once you have your food trigger diary, there are several ways you can proceed. One is to visit the doctor and ask for an allergy test. There are two main forms of testing.

Skin prick testing

A small amount of the suspected culprit is applied under the skin surface. This is done by applying a drop of the suspect allergen and then scratching the skin. Within about ten minutes, if you are allergic to that substance, the skin reacts by forming a raised, red swelling. This test can also be used to detect allergy to other factors such as house dust mites, pollens, moulds and animal dander.

If a skin prick test does prove positive, the next step is to test for specific foods by eliminating the suspected culprits from your diet. If the skin prick test proves negative, this does not prove that you are not food sensitive. Where there is a strong suspicion of a particular food, it may still be worth trying an elimination diet (see below).

Blood testing

There are several types of blood tests that measure the levels of antibodies in the blood following the ingestion of foods. The most common is the RAST test (short for radioallergosorbent test), which is also known as the IgE antibody test. This tests for levels of IgE, the antibody involved in a true allergic reaction. However, it will not detect delayed food hypersensitivity because this does not involve the production of IgE. Like the skin prick test, this test can also give a false-negative, and, practically speaking, it can only test for a small number of foods.

Other tests

You may have read about other types of testing, which are often used by complementary or alternative practitioners. These may include kinesiology, or muscle testing, hair analysis and vega testing. It has to be said that none of these has been shown scientifically to work and most orthodox doctors do not recommend them.

Dietary testing

Although the tests previously described can aid in a diagnosis of food sensitivity, the only foolproof way of detecting if food is a factor in your eczema is to follow what doctors call an exclusion or elimination diet. This is an eating regimen in which the food or foods that may potentially cause problems are avoided, and then reintroduced one by one to see if there is a flare-up of symptoms. During this time you should continue to keep your food diary and note all symptoms.

Although modified exclusion diets can sometimes be tried without supervision, any more stringent exclusion regimen should only ever be attempted under the supervision of a qualified dietitian, nutritionist or doctor with an interest in allergy. It is vital to understand that no food should ever be excluded from a child's diet without expert supervision as there is a serious danger of undernourishment.

There are many different kinds of exclusion diet, some of which are fairly simple to follow and others that are extremely rigid. Simple or modified exclusion diets involve simply leaving out the most common allergenic foods (see page 108–109). Perhaps the most popular is a diet devised by doctors in the United States and tested at the UK's Great Ormond Street Hospital for Sick Children.

More stringent exclusion diets involve consuming only a few foods for the duration of the diet, and may even involve a five-day fast. You should never fast without medical supervision. One of the most common is the lamb (or turkey) and pears diet, in which, as the name suggests, all foods are banned except lamb or turkey, peeled pears and mineral water. The idea is that because these are foods that are not usually staples, they are less often involved in food sensitivity. Another diet, sometimes called the rare foods diet, involves excluding common foods and eating only exotic foods such as yams, sweet potatoes, mangoes and papaya. If these particular foods form a normal part of your diet you should, obviously, avoid eating them.

What to expect

You need to choose a suitable time to go on an exclusion diet. It is hard, if not impossible, to embark on such a diet during a holiday or religious festival, or when there is a special occasion coming up. To make life easier, you should stock up on the foods you are allowed to eat so they are readily available. Many people find it easier at a weekend when they are less likely to be at work and have fewer commitments.

It is very common when there is a food sensitivity to experience a temporary worsening of symptoms when you first go on an exclusion diet. This should settle down over six or seven days. It is easy to become discouraged during this phase and it can be quite tough to stick with the diet. If this happens, bear in mind that experts usually regard it as a positive sign which indicates that food could indeed be a factor in your eczema. Follow your dietitian or doctor's instructions to the letter and do not stay on the diet for longer than advised.

The next phase of the diet is called the challenge, because you literally challenge your body by reintroducing the foods you have eliminated one by one to see if they cause a reaction. Once you start reintroducing foods, you may experience symptoms straight away or there may be a delayed reaction. Normally, if you have not experienced a reaction within five hours, you can assume that that particular food is not a culprit. Keep a note of any symptoms and, if a reaction occurs, take the food you have reintroduced off the menu again for two or

CAN SUPPLEMENTS HELP?

Many nutritional therapists (practitioners who specialize in treating illnesses by manipulating the diet) use food supplements as part of their treatment programme. The precise supplements prescribed will depend on your individual needs.

A common recommendation for atopic eczema would be a multi-vitamin and mineral supplement, a zinc supplement and a supplement of evening primrose oil, which is a rich source of GLA (gamma linoleic acid), found to be beneficial for some people suffering from eczema. People with atopic dermatitis may be recommended to take vegetable oils such as sunflower, safflower or linseed.

Children may be prescribed a broad multi-vitamin and mineral supplement, particularly if they are having to follow a restricted diet because of eczema made worse by food sensitivity.

Although vitamin or mineral supplements can sometimes be helpful in providing essential nutrients, it is important to recognize that they should never become a substitute for eating a healthy, well-balanced diet. We still do not know all the nutrients that food contains and many nutrients work synergistically – together – rather than one by one.

So, even if you are following an exclusion diet, enjoy your food! The next chapter contains a host of delicious recipes which will help you plan a healthy diet that contains all the nutrients you need.

three days before reintroducing another food. To make life easier, you will usually be advised to reintroduce foods that are less likely to cause a reaction first and those that are more likely to be allergenic, such as wheat and dairy foods, towards the end of the reintroduction phase. You should consume a normal-sized portion of foods you introduce as if you consume too small a portion you may not spot a positive reaction.

Dietary treatment for eczema

Once you have gone through the challenge phase, you should have two lists: one of foods that cause you problems and another of foods to which you are not sensitive. You and your professional adviser can then use this list to devise a healthy diet that includes all the nutrients you need without causing symptoms. Bear in mind the principles of healthy eating outlined on pages 100–104 and make sure that you consume a well-balanced varied diet.

After a period of time, you may be able to introduce small amounts of foods to which you are sensitive without them causing a recurrence of symptoms. However, you should not eat them on a regular basis again as symptoms are more than likely to recur.

Feeding babies and children with eczema

Because of the difficulty of identifying food sensitivities and the dangers of putting children on a restricted diet, some orthodox doctors are reluctant to try dietary treatment for eczema in children.

It is not easy following the dietary approach at the best of times, but it can be especially difficult for parents to impose dietary restrictions on a child. Just how difficult it is will depend on your child's age and temperament, the number of foods that have to be excluded and your family circumstances.

Children, especially babies and toddlers, can be notoriously fussy in their eating habits and limiting what they eat still further can, understandably, be enough to put any parent off. Older children may refuse to follow the diet or eat foods that are forbidden at other people's houses or school. Your child – and you – will need a great deal of support and encouragement if you do decide to follow a dietary approach.

Having said all this, many experts believe that in cases of severe eczema that are not being helped by other methods, diet can make a real difference and can help alleviate troublesome symptoms such as redness and scratching.

According to the UK's National Eczema Society, the children most likely to be helped by taking a dietary approach are young children (under three), babies and small children with moderate to severe eczema which is accompanied by other symptoms such as rashes, diarrhoea and a runny nose, and children who have a definite allergic reaction (immediate hypersensitivity) to consuming certain foods such as cows' milk and eggs.

Imposing a child's diet
If you do decide to try a dietary approach, the following guidelines will ensure maximum benefit.
❑ Follow the diet to the letter. Do not give your child occasional allergenic foods as this can make matters worse.
❑ Learn how to read labels; there are many baby foods and convenience foods that may contain hidden allergens such as milk, soya or cornstarch.

- ❏ Seek professional advice to ensure that your child is getting the correct nutrition for his or her age and nutritional needs.
- ❏ Make sure your child has some treats. These don't always have to be food.
- ❏ If your child is eating away from home, for instance at a party or friend's house, make sure that the person who is providing the food knows about his or her special needs. If it is not possible to avoid particular foods you may need to pack special foods for your child to take.
- ❏ Be aware that dietary treatment alone is unlikely to cure your child's eczema. You are still likely to need to use emollient therapy and topical steroids.

Which milk?

Complete breast-feeding, preferably for 4–6 months, is the best method of feeding for a newborn baby. However, after weaning, cows' milk generally forms a staple part of the diet for children. It is a valuable source of protein needed for growth and of calcium for healthy bones. So what can you feed your baby or toddler if he is sensitive to cows' milk?

You may have read that goats' milk is a suitable substitute, but this is a myth. Babies under a year should not be given goats' milk as it doesn't contain the correct balance of nutrients, and, unless it has been pasteurized, it can cause infections. Additionally, because goats' milk contains a similar protein to cows' milk, around eight out of ten children who are sensitive to cows' milk also react badly to goats' milk.

Soya milk may be a suitable substitute for some babies and children, provided that you feed a soya infant formula, which has been modified and fortified with additional nutrients, rather than soya milk in cartons, which does not contain all the nutrients they need. However, because soya is another common food trigger, it too may prove to be unsuitable.

For most babies and toddlers, the best alternative to cows' milk is often a hydrolyzed cows' milk formula, which has been processed to break down its protein, so preventing it from triggering allergic reactions. Several different products are available on prescription for atopic babies and children. Your doctor or health visitor can advise you which is the most suitable for your child.

Can diet prevent childhood eczema?

Prevention is always better than cure and research has shown that there are some definite dietary measures that may help reduce your child's risk of developing eczema, especially if you or your partner have a history of allergy or if you already have a child with an allergic condition such as eczema, asthma or hay fever.

Pregnancy matters

Although it is not necessary to eat for two, a healthy, nutritious diet is vital during pregnancy to ensure that your unborn baby grows and develops as he or she should. The rules of healthy eating outlined on pages 100–104 should be followed. You should aim to eat a varied diet and avoid eating too much of any one particular food.

Research is currently going on into whether mothers-to-be should eliminate common food triggers from their own diet during pregnancy. However, so far the results have been inconclusive. Some experts suggest that it may be worth avoiding nuts during pregnancy to help prevent your child developing a nut allergy.

Breast is best

One of the most important things you can do to help prevent your child developing eczema is to breast-feed fully for 4–6 months. That means feeding your baby breast milk alone – no top-up bottles, cereals or other food. Because breast-fed babies can sometimes be sensitive to foods in the mother's diet, there has been some discussion about whether it would be beneficial for the breast-feeding mother to avoid common food triggers such as eggs, cows' milk and fish. Again, studies have not been conclusive. The current advice is that unless your baby develops symptoms suggestive of food sensitivity – for instance eczema, 'three-month colic', sleep problems or diarrhoea – there is no benefit to be gained from limiting your own diet. If your baby does develop symptoms, seek the advice of your doctor, dietitian or health visitor before changing your diet. Again, it is worth avoiding nuts if there is a history of atopy in your family. If you can't or do not wish to breast-feed, your baby should be fed an anti-allergenic baby milk formula such as the hydrolyzed formulas that are available.

Introducing solids

As for weaning your baby onto solid foods, research has shown that babies weaned under four months are significantly more likely to develop eczema. For this reason, you should delay weaning your baby onto solids for at least four months and preferably for six. When you do start offering solids, start with foods that are least likely to trigger an allergic reaction, such as baby rice and puréed fruits and vegetables. Avoid common food triggers, such as cows' milk, eggs, wheat, peanuts, citrus fruits, chocolate and fish, until your baby is at least 6–9 months old and possibly until he is a year old.

Introduce these foods one at a time and wait a day so that you can note any adverse reactions. Because children are more easily sensitized to allergens if they have an infection or diarrhoea, avoid introducing any new foods if your child is ill. Your health visitor, doctor or dietitian can advise you on a suitable weaning regimen. Children from atopic families should never have peanut butter or other nut products before the age of three and preferably not until they are older.

NUTRIENTS FOR HEALTHY SKIN

Nutrient	Found in	Needed for
Vitamin A (beta-carotene)	Carrots, asparagus, cayenne pepper, sorrel, kale, spinach, cress, sweet potatoes, parsley, apples, garlic, ginger, papaya, rye	Repairing damaged skin and countering infections. Also helps ease symptoms of allergic reaction. Encourages moisture retention.
B complex vitamins	Rice, wheatgerm, sunflower seeds, apples, garlic, papaya, turnips, oatmeal, sesame seeds, fish, eggs, yeast, liver, kidney, almonds, parsley, watercress, sprouted seeds	Help to combat dryness and itchiness. Help relieve stress. May be especially helpful in seborrhoeic dermatitis.
Vitamin C	Oranges, apples, watercress, garlic, onions, turnips, cayenne pepper, sweet red peppers, parsley, walnuts, lemons, green leafy vegetables	Has anti-histamine effects. Helps combat skin infections.
Vitamin E	Apples, parsley, rye, wheatgerm, wholewheat, broccoli, eggs	A valuable antioxidant. Helps combat free-radical damage and protects cells.
Quercetins	Citrus fruits, green tea	Help stabilize cell membranes, so helping to block allergic response.
Zinc	Apricots, peaches, oysters, clams, cocoa, mustard seeds, eggs, pumpkin seeds	Aids healing and skin health. Shortages are found in people with eczema. These can affect metabolism of fatty acids.
Omega-3 fatty acids	Soya beans, rapeseed oil, walnuts, oily fish such as sardines, tuna, mackerel, salmon	Help reduce inflammation.
Omega-6 fatty acids	Olive oil, sunflower oil	Produce steroid-like chemicals that help control inflammation. A shortage is linked to skin problems and impaired immune response.

7 Exclusion recipes

This section presents a selection of recipes specifically designed for those people whose eczema is triggered by certain foods. It can be hard to find interesting and inspiring recipes when you have to leave out many of your favourite ingredients.

These recipes, however, show that it is still possible to create delicious, nutritious and varied meals even if you are keeping a tight control on what you eat. You'll also find on the following pages a number of recipes using foods that are rarely associated with food sensitivity, such as game. There are ideas for every kind of eating, from soups and main courses to salads and snacks.

Once you've become accustomed to the approach, you can use our recipes as a guide to help you devise other recipes which exclude foods that make your symptoms worse.

Soups and salads

Chilled pea soup

alcohol free ✓ | citrus free ✕ | dairy free ✓ | gluten free ✓ | wheat free ✓

Serves 4
Preparation time: 20 minutes, plus chilling
Cooking time: 15–20 minutes

Per serving
Energy 130 kcals/547 kJ | Protein 8 g | Carbohydrate 23 g | Fat 1 g
Fibre 8 g

375 g (12 oz) fresh shelled peas or frozen petit pois
250 g (8 oz) potatoes, chopped
1 onion, chopped
1 large mint sprig
finely grated rind and juice of ½ lemon
900 ml (1½ pints) chicken stock
salt and pepper
1 tablespoon chopped mint, to garnish

1 Put the peas into a large saucepan with the potatoes, onion, mint sprig, lemon rind and juice and stock, and season to taste with salt and pepper. Bring to the boil, then lower the heat, cover and simmer for 15–20 minutes until the peas are tender.

2 Blend in a food processor or blender, or push with a wooden spoon through a fine sieve. Set aside to cool.

3 Adjust the seasoning to taste and chill in the refrigerator for 2–3 hours. Serve chilled, sprinkled with chopped mint.

Fresh tomato soup

alcohol free ✓ | citrus free ✕ | dairy free ✓ | gluten free ✓ | wheat free ✓

Serves 8
Preparation time: 20 minutes
Cooking time: 35 minutes

Per serving
Energy 48 kcals/205 kJ | Protein 1 g | Carbohydrate 7 g | Fat 2 g
Fibre 2 g

1 tablespoon vegetable oil
1 small onion, chopped
1 kg (2 lb) ripe tomatoes, roughly chopped
1 sugar cube
1 orange
1.8 litres (3 pints) chicken or vegetable stock
2 cloves
1 bouquet garni
salt and pepper
thyme leaves, to garnish

1 Heat the oil in a large saucepan and cook the onion and tomatoes
for about 8 minutes until soft. Rub the sugar cube over the peel
of the orange to absorb the zest, and add with the remaining
ingredients to the tomato mixture. Bring to the boil, then lower
the heat, cover and simmer gently for 25 minutes. Remove the
cloves and bouquet garni.

2 Blend the soup in a food processor or blender, then push with a
wooden spoon through a fine sieve. Reheat, season to taste with
salt and pepper and serve, garnished with thyme leaves.

Chilli bean and pepper soup

alcohol free ✓ | citrus free ✗ | dairy free ✓ | gluten free ✗ | wheat free ✗

Serves 6
Preparation time: 20 minutes
Cooking time: 50 minutes

Per serving
Energy 219 kcals/918 kJ | Protein 8 g | Carbohydrate 24 g | Fat 11 g
Fibre 7 g

2 tablespoons sunflower oil
1 large onion, finely chopped
4 garlic cloves, finely chopped
2 red peppers, cored, deseeded and diced
2 red chillies, deseeded and finely chopped
900 ml (1½ pints) vegetable stock
750 ml (1¼ pints) tomato juice or passata
1 tablespoon double concentrate tomato purée
1 tablespoon sun-dried tomato paste
2 tablespoons sweet chilli sauce, or more to taste
400 g (13 oz) can red kidney beans, drained
2 tablespoons finely chopped coriander
coriander sprigs, to garnish
corn tortilla chips, to serve

Avocado Salsa:
1 firm ripe avocado
2 tablespoons lime juice
1 tablespoon finely chopped coriander
2 spring onions, finely sliced
salt and pepper

1 To make the avocado salsa, cut the avocado in half, remove the stone and peel off the skin. Cut the flesh into 1 cm (½ inch) dice and put them into a bowl with the lime juice, coriander and spring onions. Season to taste with salt and pepper and toss lightly to combine without breaking up the avocado. Cover and refrigerate until required.

2 Heat the oil in a large saucepan and fry the onion and garlic until soft but not coloured. Stir in the peppers and chillies, and fry for a few minutes. Stir in the stock and tomato juice or passata, the tomato purée and paste, chilli sauce, kidney beans and coriander. Bring to the boil, then lower the heat, cover and simmer for 30 minutes.

3 Cool slightly, then blend in a food processor or blender until smooth, or push with a wooden spoon through a fine sieve. Return to the pan and taste, adding extra chilli sauce, if necessary. Bring to the boil and serve in warmed soup bowls, topped with the avocado salsa and coriander sprigs and accompanied by tortilla chips.

Cucumber and pineapple salad with guacamole

alcohol free ✓ | citrus free ✕ | dairy free ✓ | gluten free ✓ | wheat free ✓

Serves 6
Preparation time: 20 minutes, plus standing

Per serving
Energy 178 kcals/740 kJ | Protein 2 g | Carbohydrate 14 g | Fat 13 g
Fibre: 2 g

½ cucumber, peeled and very thinly sliced
1 teaspoon salt
½ pineapple, peeled, cored and cut into bite-sized pieces
1 bunch of coriander
salt and pepper

Guacamole:
2 ripe avocados, roughly chopped
1 garlic clove, crushed
2 tablespoons lime juice
1 red chilli, finely chopped
1 tomato, finely chopped
2 spring onions, finely chopped

1 Put the cucumber slices into a colander and sprinkle with the salt. Leave to drain over a large plate or in the sink for 20–30 minutes.

2 Put the pineapple in a bowl. Roughly tear about half of the coriander leaves into the bowl.

3 Rinse the cucumber slices under cold running water. Drain thoroughly, tip on to kitchen paper to dry slightly, then add to the pineapple mixture with salt and pepper to taste. Toss lightly to mix.

4 To make the guacamole, put all the ingredients in a bowl with the remaining coriander and mash together thoroughly with a fork. Season to taste with salt and pepper. Serve immediately with the cucumber and pineapple salad.

Fiery green salad with poppadum strips

alcohol free ✓ | citrus free ✓ | dairy free ✓ | gluten free ✗ | wheat free ✗

Serves 4
Preparation time: 15 minutes, plus standing
Cooking time: 10 minutes

Per serving
Energy 181 kcals/754 kJ | Protein 6 g | Carbohydrate 11 g | Fat 14 g
Fibre 4 g

175 g (6 oz) mixed green salad leaves (e.g. little gem,
    cos, rocket, young spinach)
small handful of torn coriander leaves
2 large red chillies
4 poppadums
oil, for shallow frying
salt and pepper

Tomato, Garlic and Herb Dressing:
500 g (1 lb) ripe tomatoes, skinned, deseeded and finely diced
2 garlic cloves, finely chopped
2 tablespoons balsamic vinegar
4 tablespoons extra virgin olive oil
6 large basil leaves, finely shredded
3 tablespoons chopped mixed fresh herbs (e.g. dill, chervil,
    chives, parsley, mint)

1 First, make the dressing. Place the tomatoes in a bowl with the garlic, balsamic vinegar and olive oil. Add the shredded basil, mixed herbs and salt and pepper to taste. Mix thoroughly. Leave to stand for at least 30 minutes before using, to allow the flavours to develop.

2 Arrange the salad leaves and coriander on a large plate.

3 Cook the whole chillies under a preheated hot grill for about 5–7 minutes, turning frequently, until the skins are blistered and blackened all over. Allow to cool slightly, then carefully remove and discard the skins and seeds. Cut the flesh into thin slivers and set aside.

4 Cut the poppadums into strips about the width of a finger. Heat the oil in a frying pan and drop in the strips, a few at a time. Cook briefly (1–2 seconds only) until crisp and golden. Remove quickly from the pan and drain on kitchen paper. Serve the salad with the poppadum strips scattered over, if liked, or separately.

French bean and apricot salad

alcohol free ✓ | citrus free ✓ | dairy free ✓ | gluten free ✓ | wheat free ✓

Serves 6
Preparation time: 10 minutes
Cooking time: 5–7 minutes

Per serving
Energy 125 kcals/516 kJ | Protein 3 g | Carbohydrate 6 g | Fat 10 g
Fibre 4 g

500 g (1 lb) French beans, topped and tailed
6 ripe apricots, halved, stoned and sliced
a few parsley sprigs, roughly torn
1 tablespoon chopped tarragon
25 g (1 oz) flaked almonds, toasted, to garnish

Dressing:
4 tablespoons extra virgin olive oil
3 tablespoons white wine vinegar
salt and pepper

1 Cook the beans in a saucepan of lightly salted water for 5–7 minutes until just tender. Drain in a colander and refresh under cold running water. Drain thoroughly and leave to cool.

2 Put the beans into a salad bowl and add the sliced apricots and the herbs.

3 Whisk the dressing ingredients lightly together, add to the salad and toss well. Garnish with a sprinkling of toasted flaked almonds.

Jersey royal and celery salad

alcohol free ✓ | citrus free ✗ | dairy free ✓ | gluten free ✓ | wheat free ✓

Serves 6
Preparation time: 20 minutes
Cooking time: 12 minutes

Per serving
Energy 177 kcals/739 kJ | Protein 2 g | Carbohydrate 14 g | Fat 13 g
Fibre 2 g

500 g (1 lb) small Jersey Royal potatoes, scrubbed
6 celery sticks, with leaves if possible
75 g (3 oz) black olives
3 tablespoons capers, rinsed and drained
a few parsley sprigs, roughly chopped

Tarragon and Lemon Dressing:
3 tablespoons chopped tarragon
finely grated rind and juice of 1 lemon
6 tablespoons extra virgin olive oil
1 teaspoon coarse grain mustard
salt and pepper

1 Cook the potatoes in a saucepan of lightly salted water for about
12 minutes until just tender. Drain in a colander and refresh under
cold running water. Drain thoroughly and leave to cool.

2 Slice the celery sticks diagonally and roughly chop the leaves, if
using. Put into a bowl with the olives, capers and parsley, and add
the cooled potatoes.

3 Whisk the dressing ingredients lightly together, then add to the
salad, toss well and serve.

Smoked duck and mango salad

alcohol free ✓ | citrus free ✕ | dairy free ✕ | gluten free ✓ | wheat free ✓

Serves 4
Preparation time: 10 minutes

Per serving
Energy 368 kcals/1530 kJ | Protein 14 g | Carbohydrate 12 g | Fat 30 g
Fibre 3 g

200 g (7 oz) smoked duck breast, thinly sliced
2 small ripe mangoes, peeled, stoned and thinly sliced
2 tablespoons pomegranate seeds or redcurrants
mint leaves, to garnish

Curried Mayonnaise:
4 tablespoons mayonnaise
1 teaspoon mild, gluten-free curry paste
1 tablespoon lemon juice
salt and pepper

1 Arrange the duck, mango and pomegranate seeds or redcurrants
on 4 small serving plates.

2 Mix the mayonnaise with the curry paste and lemon juice. Season
well with salt and pepper and divide it among the 4 serving
plates. Scatter with mint leaves, to garnish.

Variation
Duck and fruit make a lovely combination. You could substitute the
pomegranate or redcurrants with cranberries or cherries, if preferred.

Grilled pepper salad

alcohol free ✓ | citrus free ✓ | dairy free ✓ | gluten free ✓ | wheat free ✓

Serves 6
Preparation time: 25 minutes
Cooking time: 20 minutes

Per serving
Energy 113 kcals/470 kJ | Protein 1 g | Carbohydrate 6 g | Fat 10 g
Fibre 3 g

2 red peppers
2 yellow peppers
2 green peppers
2 garlic cloves, chopped
1 tablespoon chopped parsley
2 basil sprigs, finely chopped
5 tablespoons extra virgin olive oil
2 teaspoons balsamic vinegar
salt and pepper
basil leaves, to garnish

1 Cook the whole peppers under a preheated hot grill, turning occasionally, until the skins are blistered and blackened all over. This will take about 20 minutes. Allow to cool slightly.

2 When cool enough to handle, hold the peppers over a bowl to catch the juices, and remove and discard the pepper skins, cores and seeds.

3 Cut the flesh into long, thin strips and arrange in a shallow serving dish. Sprinkle the chopped garlic and herbs over the top of the pepper strips and season to taste with salt and pepper.

4 Drizzle the oil and vinegar over the salad and serve, garnished with basil leaves.

Carrot and caraway salad

alcohol free ✓ | citrus free ✗ | dairy free ✓ | gluten free ✓ | wheat free ✓

Serves 4
Preparation time: 15 minutes
Cooking time: 4–5 minutes

Per serving
Energy 162 kcals/673 kJ | Protein 1 g | Carbohydrate 14 g | Fat 12 g
Fibre 3 g

500 g (1 lb) carrots
2 teaspoons caraway seeds
2 teaspoons soft light brown sugar
150 ml (¼ pint) water

Dressing:
juice of ½ orange
½ teaspoon finely grated orange rind
4 tablespoons grapeseed oil or 2 tablespoons sunflower oil plus
    2 tablespoons olive oil
salt and pepper
fresh herbs, to garnish

1 Cut the carrots into 'batons' – about 5 x 1 cm (2 x ½ inch) lengths. Put them into a medium saucepan with the caraway seeds, sugar and the water. Bring to the boil and cook, uncovered, on a fairly high heat until all the water has evaporated, stirring once or twice. This should take about 5 minutes and the carrots should be still just firm. Transfer to a shallow serving dish.

2 Meanwhile, to prepare the dressing, put the orange juice and rind into a small bowl and gradually whisk in the oil. Alternatively, shake all the ingredients together in a screw-top jar. Season well with salt and pepper.

3 Pour the orange dressing over the carrots while they are still hot. Allow to cool. Serve sprinkled with fresh herbs, to garnish.

Grilled salmon and scallop salad

alcohol free ✓ | citrus free ✗ | dairy free ✗ | gluten free ✗ | wheat free ✗

Serves 4
Preparation time: 25 minutes, plus marinating
Cooking time: 8–10 minutes

Per serving
Energy 1007 kcals/4206 kJ | Protein 62 g | Carbohydrate 55 g | Fat 61 g
Fibre 4 g

500 g (1 lb) salmon steaks
500 g (1 lb) shelled large scallops
mixed salad leaves
250 g (8 oz) conchiglie, cooked and cooled

Marinade:
150 ml (¼ pint) light olive oil
pared rind of ½ lemon
2 teaspoons chopped oregano
1 tablespoon chopped dill
salt and pepper

Dressing:
8 tablespoons mayonnaise
4 tablespoons natural yogurt

1 Mix all the marinade ingredients together and pour into a large, shallow dish. Cut the salmon into chunks equal in size to the scallops. Thread the salmon and scallops alternately on to 4 long skewers. Arrange in the marinade, turning them to coat in the flavoured oil. Leave for 1½–2 hours, turning occasionally.

2 Remove the brochettes from the marinade, reserving the marinade, and arrange in one layer on a grill rack. Cook under a preheated hot grill for 8–10 minutes, turning frequently and basting with the reserved marinade.

3 Meanwhile, stir together the mayonnaise and yogurt and set aside. Arrange a bed of salad leaves and cooked pasta on 4 serving plates.

4 To serve, remove the seafood from the skewers and pile on to the salad. Serve the dressing separately.

Vegetable dishes

Pumpkin curry

alcohol free ✓ | citrus free ✓ | dairy free ✓ | gluten free ✓ | wheat free ✓

Serves 6
Preparation time: 20 minutes, plus soaking
Cooking time: 30–35 minutes

Per serving
Energy 105 kcals/437 kJ | Protein 2 g | Carbohydrate 8 g | Fat 7 g
Fibre 3 g

50 g (2 oz) fresh coconut, grated
300 ml (½ pint) coconut water (from a fresh coconut)
2 tablespoons vegetable oil
1 onion, chopped
1 green pepper, cored, deseeded and chopped
4 garlic cloves, crushed
2 slices of fresh root ginger, peeled and finely chopped
¼ teaspoon turmeric
2 green chillies, deseeded and finely chopped
¼ teaspoon ground cloves
¼ teaspoon dried chilli flakes
750 g (1½ lb) pumpkin, peeled, deseeded and cut into
    2.5 cm (1 inch) cubes
2 tomatoes, skinned and chopped
salt and pepper

1 Put the grated coconut into a bowl and add the coconut water. You can drain this out of a fresh coconut by piercing it a couple of times with a skewer and draining out the liquid. (If you don't get enough liquid, simply make up the quantity with water.) Leave to soak for about 30 minutes.

2 Heat the oil in a large, heavy-based saucepan and fry the onion, green pepper and garlic gently over a very low heat, stirring from time to time, until the onion and pepper are soft and golden brown.

3 Add the ginger, turmeric, chillies, cloves and chilli flakes, stir well and cook over a low heat for 2–3 minutes, stirring constantly.

4 Add the pumpkin, tomatoes and the coconut mixture. Bring to the boil, then lower the heat to a bare simmer, cover and cook gently for 20 minutes until the pumpkin is tender but not mushy. Season to taste with salt and pepper and serve hot.

Spicy roasted vegetables

alcohol free ✓ | citrus free ✕ | dairy free ✓ | gluten free ✓ | wheat free ✓

Serves 6
Preparation time: 25 minutes
Cooking time: 10–12 minutes

Per serving
Energy 89 kcals/370 kJ | Protein 3 g | Carbohydrate 11 g | Fat 5 g
Fibre 4 g

2 tablespoons extra virgin olive oil
½ teaspoon white cumin seeds
1 green pepper, cored, deseeded and thickly sliced
1 red pepper, cored, deseeded and thickly sliced
1 orange pepper, cored, deseeded and thickly sliced
2 courgettes, diagonally sliced
2 tomatoes, halved
2 red onions, quartered
1 aubergine, thickly sliced
2 thick green chillies, sliced
4 garlic cloves
2.5 cm (1 inch) piece of fresh root ginger, shredded
1 teaspoon dried chilli flakes
½ teaspoon salt
1 tablespoon chopped coriander, to garnish
lemon wedges, to serve

1 Heat a grill pan under a preheated hot grill for about 2 minutes. Pour in the oil, then add the cumin seeds to the pan. Lower the heat to moderate.

2 Using a pair of tongs, arrange the vegetables in the pan, then scatter over the chillies, garlic, ginger, chilli flakes and salt. Increase the heat and cook the vegetables for 7–10 minutes, turning occasionally with the tongs.

3 Garnish with coriander and serve hot with lemon wedges.

Navarin of spring vegetables

alcohol free ✓ | citrus free ✗ | dairy free ✗ | gluten free ✓ | wheat free ✓

Serves 4
Preparation time: 20–25 minutes
Cooking time: about 25 minutes

Per serving
Energy 267 kcals/1109 kJ | Protein 9 g | Carbohydrate 21 g | Fat 17 g
Fibre 7 g

250 g (8 oz) small, shelled broad beans
175 g (6 oz) mangetout
175 g (6 oz) fine asparagus, cut into 2.5 cm (1 inch) pieces
75 g (3 oz) butter
8 spring onions, thinly sliced
2 garlic cloves, chopped
900 ml (1½ pints) vegetable stock
1 thyme sprig
15 baby onions
10 baby turnips, or 3 small turnips cut into wedges
250 g (8 oz) baby carrots
1½ tablespoons lemon juice
salt and pepper
chervil sprigs, to garnish

1 Blanch the broad beans, mangetout and asparagus separately in salted boiling water for 1 minute each. Drain in a colander and refresh immediately under cold running water. Drain thoroughly and set aside.

2 Melt the butter in a large, heavy-based pan and fry the spring onions and garlic gently until soft but not coloured. Add the stock and thyme, bring to the boil, then add the baby onions. Lower the heat, cover and simmer for 5 minutes.

3 Add the turnips, bring back to the boil, then lower the heat and simmer for 6-8 minutes. Add the carrots and cook for 5-6 minutes. Season to taste with salt and pepper and stir in the lemon juice. Add the blanched vegetables and heat through. Serve in warmed bowls, garnished with chervil sprigs.

Stir-fried vegetables

alcohol free ✓ | citrus free ✓ | dairy free ✓ | gluten free ✓ | wheat free ✓

Serves 4
Preparation time: 15–20 minutes
Cooking time: 3–5 minutes

Per serving
Energy 60 kcals/253 kJ | Protein 3 g | Carbohydrate 6 g | Fat 3 g
Fibre 3 g

1 tablespoon vegetable oil
125 g (4 oz) bamboo shoots, thinly sliced
50 g (2 oz) mangetout
125 g (4 oz) carrots, thinly sliced
50 g (2 oz) broccoli florets
125 g (4 oz) bean sprouts
1 teaspoon salt
1 teaspoon sugar
1 tablespoon stock or water

1 Heat the oil in a wok or large frying pan and add the bamboo shoots, mangetout, carrots and broccoli florets. Stir-fry for about 1 minute.

2 Add the bean sprouts with the salt and sugar. Stir-fry for a further minute or so, then add the stock or water. Do not overcook or the vegetables will lose their crunchiness. Serve immediately.

Artichokes provençal

alcohol free ✓ | citrus free ✗ | dairy free ✓ | gluten free ✓ | wheat free ✓

Serves 6
Preparation time: 20 minutes
Cooking time: 30 minutes

Per serving
Energy 93 kcals/452 kJ | Protein 4 g | Carbohydrate 22 g | Fat 1 g
Fibre 1 g

1 kg (2 lb) Jerusalem artichokes, scraped
2 large garlic cloves, crushed
500 g (1 lb) tomatoes, peeled, deseeded and chopped
2 tablespoons tomato purée
2 tablespoons lemon juice
1 tablespoon chopped basil
1 teaspoon sugar
salt and pepper
2 tablespoons chopped parsley, to garnish

1 Slice the artichokes thickly and steam or poach them in lightly
salted water for about 20 minutes until tender.

2 Meanwhile, mix the garlic and the tomatoes in a saucepan and
cook over a moderate heat for about 10 minutes, stirring
frequently, until the liquid has reduced a little.

3 When the texture is pulpy, add the tomato purée, lemon juice,
basil, sugar and salt and pepper to taste. Heat through and pour
over the cooked artichokes in a serving dish. Sprinkle with
chopped parsley, to garnish. This dish is equally delicious served
hot or cold.

Ratatouille niçoise

alcohol free ✓ | citrus free ✓ | dairy free ✓ | gluten free ✓ | wheat free ✓

Serves 6
Preparation time: 20 minutes
Cooking time: 40 minutes

Per serving
Energy 237 kcals/985 kJ | Protein 5 g | Carbohydrate 19 g | Fat 17 g
Fibre 6 g

125 ml (4 fl oz) olive oil
500 g (1 lb) aubergines, thinly sliced
500 g (1 lb) courgettes, sliced
500 g (1 lb) red onions, thinly sliced
500 g (1 lb) green peppers, cored, deseeded and thinly sliced
5 garlic cloves, crushed
750 g (1½ lb) tomatoes, skinned and roughly chopped
2 thyme sprigs
5 basil leaves
salt and pepper
chopped parsley, to garnish

1 Heat half of the oil in a large saucepan and fry the aubergines gently over a moderate heat, stirring frequently, until they are lightly golden.

2 Add the courgettes and continue frying for 5–6 minutes until lightly coloured. Remove the vegetables from the pan with a slotted spoon and set aside.

3 Add the remaining oil to the pan and fry the onions gently until soft and golden. Add the peppers and garlic, increase the heat and fry for 3–4 minutes. Add the chopped tomatoes and cook gently for 10 minutes. Stir in the aubergines and courgettes, season to taste with salt and pepper and crumble in the thyme. Cook gently, uncovered, for about 20 minutes. Tear the basil leaves into the ratatouille, and serve it warm or cold, sprinkled with parsley, to garnish.

Grilled asparagus salad

alcohol free ✓ | citrus free ✗ | dairy free ✓ | gluten free ✓ | wheat free ✓

Serves 4
Preparation time: 15 minutes
Cooking time: 7 minutes

Per serving
Energy 258 kcals/1063 kJ | Protein 4 g | Carbohydrate 4 g | Fat 25 g
Fibre 2 g

500 g (1 lb) asparagus
3 tablespoons olive oil
about 50 g (2 oz) rocket
about 50 g (2 oz) lamb's lettuce
2 spring onions, finely chopped
3–4 radishes, thinly sliced
6 tablespoons Tarragon and Lemon dressing (see page 131)
salt and pepper

To Garnish:
roughly chopped fresh herbs (e.g. tarragon, parsley, chervil, dill)
thin strips of lemon rind

1 Trim the asparagus and use a potato peeler to peel about 5 cm (2 inches) off the base of each stalk. Arrange in a single layer on a baking sheet and brush with oil. Cook under a preheated hot grill for about 7 minutes, turning frequently, until the spears are just tender when pierced with the point of a knife. Sprinkle with salt and pepper to taste and leave to cool.

2 Arrange the rocket and lamb's lettuce on a serving platter. Scatter over the spring onions and radishes.

3 Arrange the asparagus beside the salad leaves and drizzle with the dressing. Garnish with a sprinkling of herbs and thin strips of lemon rind.

Beetroot risotto

alcohol free ✓ | citrus free ✓ | dairy free ✕ | gluten free ✓ | wheat free ✓

Serves 4
Preparation time: 15 minutes
Cooking time: about 25 minutes

Per serving
Energy 780 kcals/3279 kJ | Protein 13 g | Carbohydrate 119 g | Fat 32 g
Fibre 5 g

1 tablespoon olive oil
15 g (½ oz) butter
1 teaspoon crushed coriander seeds
4 spring onions, thinly sliced
400 g (13 oz) freshly cooked beetroot, cut into 1 cm (½ inch) dice
500 g (1 lb) arborio rice
1.5 litres (2½ pints) hot vegetable stock
200 g (7 oz) cream cheese
4 tablespoons finely chopped dill
salt and pepper

To Garnish:
dill sprigs
a little crème fraîche

1 Heat the oil and butter in a large, heavy-based saucepan and stir-fry the coriander seeds and spring onions quickly for 1 minute.

2 Add the beetroot and the rice. Cook, stirring, for 2–3 minutes to coat all the grains with oil and butter. Gradually add the hot stock, a ladleful at a time, cooking and stirring frequently until each ladleful has been absorbed before adding the next. This should take about 20 minutes, by which time the rice should be tender, but still firm to the bite.

3 Stir in the cream cheese and dill, and season to taste with salt and pepper. Serve immediately, garnished with dill sprigs and a little crème fraîche.

Brown rice with mixed herbs

alcohol free ✓ | citrus free ✓ | dairy free ✓ | gluten free ✓ | wheat free ✓

Serves 4
Preparation time: 20 minutes
Cooking time: 30–35 minutes

Per serving
Energy 190 kcals/802 kJ | Protein 4 g | Carbohydrate 33 g | Fat 6 g
Fibre 2 g

1 small onion, finely chopped
1 garlic clove, finely chopped
½ teaspoon garam masala
150 g (5 oz) long-grain brown rice
pinch of powdered saffron
400 ml (14 fl oz) vegetable stock
½ tablespoon desiccated coconut
2 teaspoons olive oil
2 tablespoons tarragon vinegar
1 tablespoon chopped coriander
2 tablespoons chopped parsley
10 cashew nuts, lightly toasted
salt and pepper

1 Heat a large, heavy-based saucepan and dry-fry the onion gently for 3 minutes. Add the garlic, garam masala and rice, and fry gently for a further 2 minutes, stirring constantly.

2 Stir in the saffron, stock and coconut, and season to taste with salt and pepper. Bring to the boil, then lower the heat and simmer gently for about 25 minutes until the rice is tender.

3 Mix the oil with the vinegar and herbs, then season to taste with salt and pepper. Stir evenly through the warm rice, together with the cashew nuts.

4 Serve warm as a main course or accompaniment, or cold as a rice salad.

Chickpea and tomato rice

alcohol free ✓ | citrus free ✓ | dairy free ✕ | gluten free ✓ | wheat free ✓

Serves 6
Preparation time: 15 minutes, including standing
Cooking time: 15–20 minutes

Per serving
Energy 372 kcals/1558 kJ | Protein 11 g | Carbohydrate 70 g | Fat 6 g
Fibre 1 g

1 tablespoon ghee or butter
1 teaspoon corn oil
2 onions, sliced
2 black cardamoms
1 cinnamon stick
2 whole cloves
4 black peppercorns
1 teaspoon finely grated fresh root ginger
1 teaspoon crushed garlic
1½ teaspoons salt
2 tomatoes, sliced
425 g (14 oz) can chickpeas, drained
400 g (13 oz) basmati rice, washed and drained
2 tablespoons chopped fresh coriander
750 ml (1¼ pints) water

1 Heat the ghee or butter with the oil in a saucepan until hot. Add the onions, cardamoms, cinnamon, cloves and peppercorns and stir-fry over a high heat for about 2 minutes, then add the ginger, garlic, salt and tomatoes.

2 Stir in the drained chickpeas and rice and lower the heat to medium. Add half of the coriander. Pour in the water, cover tightly and cook for about 15–20 minutes or until all the water has been fully absorbed.

3 Remove from the heat and leave to stand for 3–5 minutes before serving the rice, garnished with the remaining coriander.

Meat and poultry

Honey duck breasts with plum and mango salsa

alcohol free ✓ | citrus free ✗ | dairy free ✓ | gluten free ✓ | wheat free ✓

Serves 4
Preparation time: 20 minutes
Cooking time: 12–15 minutes

Per serving
Energy 738 kcals/3060 kJ | Protein 32 g | Carbohydrate 19 g | Fat 60 g
Fibre 3 g

4 duck breasts, about 175 g (6 oz) each
2 tablespoons Tamari (wheat-free soy sauce)
1 tablespoon clear honey
1 teaspoon grated fresh root ginger
1 teaspoon chilli powder

Plum and Mango Salsa:
1 large ripe mango, peeled, stoned and finely diced
6–8 plums, stoned and finely diced
grated rind and juice of 1 lime
1 small red onion, finely chopped
1 tablespoon olive oil
1 tablespoon coarsely chopped mint leaves
1 tablespoon coarsely chopped coriander
salt and pepper

1 Use a sharp knife to score the duck skin lightly, cutting down into the fat but not through the meat.

2 Heat a frying pan until very hot, then lay the duck breasts in it, skin side down, and cook for 3 minutes until sealed and browned. Turn the breasts over and cook for 2 minutes. Transfer to a baking sheet, arranging them skin side up.

3 Mix the Tamari, honey, ginger and chilli powder in a small bowl. Spoon this mixture over the duck and cook in a preheated oven at 200°C (400°F), Gas Mark 6, for 6–9 minutes until cooked to your liking. The duck may be served pink or well done.

4 Meanwhile, combine all the ingredients for the salsa in a bowl and season well with salt and pepper.

5 Thinly slice the duck and fan out the slices on individual plates. Spoon some of the salsa over the duck and serve immediately, offering the remaining salsa separately.

Turkey and parma ham kebabs

alcohol free ✓ | citrus free ✕ | dairy free ✓ | gluten free ✓ | wheat free ✓

Serves 4
Preparation time: 20 minutes, plus marinating
Cooking time: 8–10 minutes

Per serving
Energy 225 kcals/949 kJ | Protein 36 g | Carbohydrate 2 g | Fat 8 g
Fibre 1 g

500 g (1 lb) turkey fillet, cut into 4 cm (1½ inch) cubes
grated rind of 1 lemon
1 small onion, finely chopped
1 garlic clove, finely chopped
2 tablespoons chopped basil
2 teaspoons olive oil
125 g (4 oz) Parma ham, cut into long strips
8 small button mushrooms
8 small bay leaves
8 lemon wedges
salt and pepper

1 Put the turkey into a shallow dish. Add the lemon rind with the onion, garlic, basil and oil, and season to taste with salt and pepper. Stir, cover and chill for 3–4 hours.

2 Drain the turkey, reserving the marinade. Wrap each piece of turkey in a strip of Parma ham. Thread the turkey and ham rolls on to 4 kebab skewers, alternating with the mushrooms, bay leaves and lemon wedges.

3 Brush with the marinade and cook under a preheated moderate grill for 8–10 minutes, turning halfway through and brushing with the marinade. Serve hot.

Pesto chicken kebabs

alcohol free ✓ | citrus free ✕ | dairy free ✕ | gluten free ✓ | wheat free ✓

Serves 4
Preparation time: 20 minutes
Cooking time: 12 minutes

Per serving
Energy 524 kcals/2180 kJ | Protein 44 g | Carbohydrate 2 g | Fat 38 g
Fibre 0 g

4 chicken breast fillets, about 125 g (4 oz) each
2 tablespoons pesto
8 slices of Parma ham
125 g (4 oz) sun-dried tomatoes in oil, finely chopped
125 g (4 oz) mozzarella cheese, finely diced
1 tablespoon olive oil
salt and pepper
chopped parsley, to garnish
lemon wedges, to serve

1 Place a chicken fillet between 2 sheets of clingfilm and pound lightly with a mallet until it is about 1 cm (½ inch) thick. Repeat with the remaining fillets.

2 Spread pesto over each chicken fillet and lay 2 slices of Parma ham on top. Sprinkle the tomatoes and mozzarella evenly over the chicken, then season to taste with salt and pepper. Roll up each fillet and cut the rolls into 2.5 cm (1 inch) slices. Thread the slices on to 4 metal skewers.

3 Brush the rolls lightly with oil and cook them under a preheated moderate grill for about 6 minutes on each side until cooked through and brown on the outside. Garnish with chopped parsley, and serve hot with the lemon wedges.

Marinated lamb kebabs

alcohol free ✓ | citrus free ✗ | dairy free ✗ | gluten free ✓ | wheat free ✓

Serves 4
Preparation time: 30 minutes, plus marinating
Cooking time: 10–15 minutes

Per serving
Energy 127 kcals/530 kJ | Protein 14 g | Carbohydrate 7 g | Fat 5 g
Fibre 2 g

200 g (7 oz) boneless lamb, cut into fine strips
4 small tomatoes, halved
125 g (4 oz) button mushrooms
1 green pepper, cored, deseeded and cut into 2.5 cm (1 inch) cubes
8 bay leaves

Marinade:
150 ml (¼ pint) low-fat natural yogurt
4 tablespoons lemon juice
2 teaspoons salt
1 teaspoon pepper
1 small onion, grated

To Serve:
boiled rice
salad

1 Mix together all the marinade ingredients in a bowl. Place the meat in the marinade and leave for approximately 24 hours, turning occasionally.

2 Reserve the marinade and thread the strips of meat on to 4 long or 8 short skewers, alternating with the tomatoes, mushrooms, green pepper and the bay leaves.

3 Cook under a preheated hot grill, turning once, for 10–15 minutes. Brush the vegetables with the marinade once or twice during cooking, to prevent them drying out. Serve with boiled rice and salad.

Lamb shanks with olives, sun-dried tomatoes and saffron mash

alcohol free ✕ | citrus free ✓ | dairy free ✕ | gluten free ✕ | wheat free ✕

Serves 4
Preparation time: 25 minutes
Cooking time: 2–2½ hours

Per serving
Energy 763 kcals/3185 kJ | Protein 33 g | Carbohydrate 60 g | Fat 41 g
Fibre 6 g

4 lamb shanks, about 500 g (1 lb) each
2 tablespoons plain flour
2 tablespoons olive oil
2 red onions, sliced
2 tablespoons rosemary leaves
3 garlic cloves, chopped
100 ml (3½ fl oz) balsamic vinegar
200 ml (7 fl oz) red wine
50 g (2 oz) pitted black olives, quartered
40 g (1½ oz) sun-dried tomatoes, cut into strips
175 ml (6 fl oz) water
salt and pepper

Saffron Mash:
1 kg (2 lb) potatoes, cut into large chunks
100 ml (3½ fl oz) single cream
large pinch of saffron threads
5 tablespoons extra virgin olive oil

1 Toss the lamb in the flour, shaking off any excess. Heat the oil in a heavy-based pan, large enough to hold the lamb shanks in one layer, over a moderate heat. Add the lamb and brown all over. Remove and set aside.

2 Lower the heat and cook the onions for about 10 minutes until soft. Add the rosemary and garlic and cook for a further 2–3 minutes. Increase the heat, add the vinegar and wine and boil rapidly until reduced by half. Stir in the olives, tomatoes and water. Reduce the heat and place the lamb shanks on top of the sauce. Cover with a well-fitting lid and cook for 1½–2 hours until very tender. Baste occasionally and add more water, if necessary. Season to taste with salt and pepper.

3 Meanwhile, to make the saffron mash, boil the potatoes for about 20 minutes until just tender. Heat the cream in a small pan, remove from the heat and stir in the saffron. Leave to infuse for 10 minutes. When the potatoes are cooked, drain well, return to the pan and add the saffron cream and the oil. Mash together thoroughly and season to taste with salt and pepper.

4 To serve, divide the saffron mash between 4 plates, top with the lamb shanks and spoon over some sauce.

Noisettes of lamb with savoury butter

alcohol free ✓ | citrus free ✓ | dairy free ✗ | gluten free ✓ | wheat free ✓

Serves 4
Preparation time: 25 minutes, plus freezing
Cooking time: 10 minutes

Per serving
Energy 280 kcals/1166 kJ | Protein 24 g | Carbohydrate 0 g | Fat 20 g
Fibre 1 g

8 lamb noisettes or boneless loin chops
a few rosemary sprigs, roughly chopped, plus extra to garnish
50 g (2 oz) butter
1 garlic clove, crushed
1 tablespoon chopped parsley
salt and pepper
roasted red and yellow peppers, to serve

1 Season the lamb with a little salt and pepper and sprinkle
generously with chopped rosemary.

2 To make the savoury butter, beat the butter in a bowl until pale
and creamy. Beat in the garlic, parsley and salt and pepper to
taste. Turn out on to a sheet of greaseproof paper and, with wet
hands, work the butter back and forth to form a roll. Wrap in the
paper and freeze for about 30 minutes.

3 Cook the noisettes under a preheated hot grill for about
5 minutes, then remove from the heat. Turn the noisettes over,
top each with a slice of savoury butter and grill for a further
5 minutes. Garnish with rosemary sprigs and serve with roasted
red and yellow peppers.

Lamb and vegetable hotpot

alcohol free ✓ | citrus free ✓ | dairy free ✓ | gluten free ✓ | wheat free ✓

Serves 3
Preparation time: 20 minutes
Cooking time: 45 minutes

Per serving
Energy 177 kcals/740 kJ | Protein 19 g | Carbohydrate 13 g | Fat 6 g
Fibre 5 g

150 g (5 oz) lean cooked lamb, cut into cubes
75 g (3 oz) leeks, sliced
125 g (4 oz) cauliflower, broken into florets
50 g (2 oz) mushrooms, sliced
200 g (7 oz) carrots, sliced
1 onion, sliced
2 tomatoes, sliced
150 ml (¼ pint) vegetable stock
salt and freshly ground black pepper
broad beans, to serve (optional)

1 Remove any fat from the meat. Arrange the meat and vegetables, except the tomatoes, in layers in a casserole. Sprinkle with salt and pepper to taste, then arrange the tomato slices over the top. Pour in the vegetable stock and cover.

2 Cook in the centre of a preheated oven at 180°C (350°F), Gas Mark 4, for 45 minutes. Serve hot with broad beans, if liked.

Spicy pork rolls with minted yogurt

alcohol free ✓ | citrus free ✕ | dairy free ✕ | gluten free ✓ | wheat free ✓

Serves 4
Preparation time: 20 minutes
Cooking time: 10–12 minutes

Per serving
Energy 260 kcals/1086 kJ | Protein 30 g | Carbohydrate 5 g | Fat 14 g
Fibre 0 g

4 pork escalopes, about 125 g (4 oz) each
1 small onion, coarsely chopped
1 red chilli, deseeded and coarsely chopped
4 tablespoons coarsely chopped fresh coriander
grated rind and juice of 1 lime
1 tablespoon Thai fish sauce
2 garlic cloves, crushed
1 teaspoon grated fresh root ginger
1 teaspoon ground cumin
½ teaspoon ground coriander
50 ml (2 fl oz) coconut milk
mint leaves, to garnish

Minted Yogurt:
4 tablespoons coarsely chopped mint leaves
200 ml (7 fl oz) Greek yogurt
salt and pepper

1 Lay a pork escalope between 2 sheets of clingfilm and beat it out with a mallet to a thickness of 5 mm (¼ inch). Repeat with the remaining escalopes.

2 Blend the remaining ingredients to a coarse paste in a food processor or blender. Spread a quarter of the paste over a thin pork escalope and roll up to enclose the filling. Secure the roll with a wooden cocktail stick. Repeat with the remaining paste and pork.

3 Place the pork rolls on a baking sheet and cook in a preheated oven at 200°C (400°F), Gas Mark 6, for about 10–12 minutes until cooked through.

4 Stir the mint into the yogurt and add salt and pepper to taste. Serve the rolls hot, garnished with mint leaves, with a spoonful of the minted yogurt on the side.

Variation
These spicy rolls are equally tasty using chicken breast fillets instead of the pork. Use the same quantity.

Paella with rabbit and chicken

alcohol free ✓ | citrus free ✓ | dairy free ✓ | gluten free ✓ | wheat free ✓

Serves 4
Preparation time: about 40 minutes
Cooking time: about 1¼ hours

Per serving
Energy 966 kcals/4048 kJ | Protein 51 g | Carbohydrate 99 g | Fat 44 g
Fibre 6 g

4 tablespoons olive oil
1 kg (2 lb) chicken, cut into small pieces
4 small rabbit portions
2 Spanish onions, chopped
4 garlic cloves, chopped
1 tablespoon paprika
375 g (12 oz) paella or long-grain rice
3 large ripe tomatoes, skinned, deseeded and chopped
1.8 litres (3 pints) hot chicken stock
1 rosemary sprig
large pinch of saffron threads, crushed
150 g (5 oz) green beans, cut into short lengths
125 g (4 oz) broad beans
salt and pepper

1 Heat the oil in a casserole. Add the chicken and rabbit and cook until lightly browned. Stir in the onion and garlic. Fry for 5 minutes, then stir in the paprika and rice.

2 Stir for 2–3 minutes, then add the tomatoes with all but 2 tablespoons of the chicken stock, the rosemary and salt and pepper. Dissolve the saffron in the reserved stock, then add to the paella and boil for 8–10 minutes.

3 Scatter the green and broad beans over the paella – do not stir. Gradually turn down the heat and simmer until the rice is tender and the liquid is absorbed, about 8–10 minutes. Cover the paella with a thick cloth, remove from the heat and leave for 8 minutes before serving.

Rabbit with rosemary and mustard

alcohol free ✕ | citrus free ✓ | dairy free ✕ | gluten free ✓ | wheat free ✓

Serves 4
Preparation time: about 10 minutes
Cooking time: about 55 minutes

Per serving
Energy 215 kcals/900 kJ | Protein 25 g | Carbohydrate 6 g | Fat 7 g
Fibre 1 g

1 teaspoon olive oil
1 medium onion, finely chopped
4 rabbit joints, about 200 g (7 oz) each
300 ml (½ pint) chicken stock
200 ml (7 fl oz) dry white wine
2 teaspoons coarse grain mustard
1 tablespoon chopped rosemary, plus extra to garnish
3 tablespoons low-fat fromage frais
1 egg yolk
salt and pepper

1 Heat the oil in a large, heavy-based saucepan and fry the onion gently for 3 minutes. Add the rabbit joints and brown evenly.

2 Add the chicken stock, wine, mustard, rosemary and salt and pepper to taste. Cover and simmer for 45 minutes until the rabbit is just tender.

3 Transfer the rabbit joints with a slotted spoon to a serving dish and keep warm. Boil the cooking liquid rapidly until reduced by half. Beat the fromage frais with the egg yolk and whisk into the cooking liquid over a gentle heat, being careful not to boil it.

4 Spoon the sauce over the rabbit and garnish with chopped rosemary. Serve immediately.

8 Healthy eating

All of us – with or without skin problems – should aim to eat a healthy, nutritious diet. However, this is especially important when you have eczema because a healthy diet can play an important part in boosting your immune system, which will make you feel more energetic and may also improve your skin.

This chapter contains a selection of low-fat, tasty recipes, which are specially designed to keep you healthy and boost your immune system. They are featured because they offer a rich source of the antioxidant vitamins A, C and E, which are so important for helping to boost immunity. They are also rich in a whole host of other nutrients that are known to be especially beneficial for the skin, such as B complex vitamins, quercetins, zinc and the vital omega-3 and omega-6 fatty acids found in nuts, seeds and oily fish.

Soups and salads

Celeriac and apple soup

alcohol free ✓ | citrus free ✓ | dairy free ✗ | gluten free ✓ | wheat free ✓

Serves 6
Preparation time: 15 minutes
Cooking time: about 35 minutes

Per serving
Energy 78 kcals/325 kJ | Protein 2 g | Carbohydrate 9 g | Fat 4 g
Fibre 6 g

25 g (1 oz) butter or margarine
500 g (1 lb) celeriac, peeled and chopped
3 dessert apples, peeled, cored and chopped
1.2 litres (2 pints) chicken or vegetable stock
pinch of cayenne pepper
salt and white pepper

To Garnish:
2–3 tablespoons finely diced dessert apple
paprika

1 Melt the butter or margarine in a large saucepan and cook the celeriac and apples over a moderate heat for about 5 minutes until they have begun to soften.

2 Add the stock and cayenne pepper and bring to the boil. Lower the heat, cover and simmer for 25–30 minutes until the celeriac and apples are very soft.

3 Blend the mixture in batches in a food processor or blender until it is very smooth, transferring each successive batch to a clean saucepan. Alternatively, push with a wooden spoon through a fine sieve. Reheat gently. Season to taste with salt and pepper. Serve hot in warmed soup bowls or plates. Garnish each portion with a little finely diced apple and a dusting of paprika.

Italian leek and pumpkin soup

alcohol free ✓ | citrus free ✓ | dairy free ✗ | gluten free ✓ | wheat free ✓

Serves 8
Preparation time: 25 minutes
Cooking time: about 55 minutes

Per serving
Energy 100 kcals/428 kJ | Protein 6 g | Carbohydrate 19 g | Fat 1 g
Fibre 2 g

600 ml (1 pint) hot chicken or vegetable stock
1 Spanish onion, chopped
50 g (2 oz) leek, chopped
500 g (1 lb) pumpkin, diced
250 g (8 oz) potatoes, diced
600 ml (1 pint) skimmed milk
125 g (4 oz) cooked long-grain rice
150 ml (¼ pint) low-fat natural yogurt
salt and pepper
chopped parsley, to garnish

1 Put 2 tablespoons of the stock with the onion and leek into a large saucepan and cook over a moderate heat until soft. Add the pumpkin, potatoes, milk and remaining stock, and season to taste with salt and pepper. Bring to the boil, then lower the heat, cover and simmer for 45 minutes, stirring frequently.

2 Blend the soup in a food processor or blender, or push with a wooden spoon through a fine sieve. Return to the pan and add the cooked rice and most of the yogurt. Reheat gently. Serve topped with the remaining yogurt and sprinkled with parsley.

Jamaican pepperpot soup

alcohol free ✓ | citrus free ✓ | dairy free ✓ | gluten free ✓ | wheat free ✓

Serves 6–8
Preparation time: 30–35 minutes
Cooking time: 1¼ hour

Per serving
Energy 352 kcals/1483 kJ | Protein 40 g | Carbohydrate 26 g | Fat 11 g
Fibre 11 g

500 g (1 lb) lean stewing beef, cut into small cubes
125 g (4 oz) lean pork, cut into small cubes
1.2 litres (2 pints) water
12 okra, trimmed and chopped
250 g (8 oz) kale, chopped
1 green pepper, cored, deseeded and chopped
250 g (8 oz) spinach, chopped
1 spring onion, chopped
1 thyme sprig
¼ teaspoon cayenne pepper
250 g (8 oz) yellow yams, thinly sliced
1 small potato, thinly sliced
1 garlic clove, finely chopped
salt

1 Put the beef and pork with the water into a large saucepan. Bring
to the boil, then simmer, partially covered, for about 30 minutes.

2 Add the okra, kale, green pepper, spinach and spring onion with
the thyme and cayenne pepper. Cook over a moderate heat,
partially covered, for 15 minutes. Add the yams, potato and garlic
and cook for a further 20 minutes until soft. Add more water if
the soup is too thick. Season to taste with salt and serve in bowls.

Hearty bean soup

alcohol free ✓ | citrus free ✓ | dairy free ✕ | gluten free ✓ | wheat free ✓

Serves 6
Preparation time: 20 minutes
Cooking time: 45 minutes

Per serving
Energy 249 kcals/1050 kJ | Protein 13 g | Carbohydrate 41 g | Fat 5 g
Fibre 13 g

1 celery stick, chopped
1 large carrot, chopped
1 large onion, chopped
2 x 425 g (14 oz) cans red kidney beans
1 tablespoon olive oil
400 g (13 oz) can chopped tomatoes
2 tablespoons chopped flat leaf parsley
2 garlic cloves, chopped
½–1 teaspoon chopped rosemary
600– 900 ml (1–1½ pints) hot chicken stock or water
75 g (3 oz) arborio rice
salt and pepper
25–40 g (1–1½ oz) Parmesan cheese, freshly grated, to serve
rosemary sprigs, to garnish

1 Put the celery, carrot and onion into a heavy-based saucepan, just cover with water and simmer for 15 minutes. Add the drained beans, reserving 4–6 tablespoons. Pour the vegetables and liquid into a bowl and set aside.

2 Heat the oil in the pan and cook the tomatoes, parsley and garlic gently until the mixture thickens. Add the rosemary and salt and pepper to taste. Add the beans and vegetables with their liquid, and cook for about 5 minutes until tender. Blend in a food processor or blender, in batches if necessary, or push with a wooden spoon through a fine sieve.

3 Make up the purée to 1.5 litres (2½ pints) with stock or water. Season to taste with salt and pepper. Return to the pan and add the rice. Bring to the boil, then lower the heat and simmer for 15–20 minutes until the rice is cooked. Add the reserved beans and a little water, if necessary – this should be a very thick soup. Heat through, then sprinkle with the Parmesan and garnish with rosemary sprigs.

Rice noodle soup

alcohol free ✓ | citrus free ✗ | dairy free ✓ | gluten free ✗ | wheat free ✗

Serves 4
Preparation time: 20 minutes, plus soaking
Cooking time: 8 minutes

Per serving
Energy 217 kcals/910 kJ | Protein 7 g | Carbohydrate 42 g | Fat 2 g
Fibre 1 g

750 ml (1¼ pints) vegetable stock
3 spring onions, cut into 2.5 cm (1 inch) lengths
2 baby corns, obliquely sliced
1 tomato, quartered
1 onion, cut into 8 pieces
6 kaffir lime leaves, finely chopped
1 celery stick, chopped
125 g (4 oz) ready-steamed tofu, diced
1 tablespoon soy sauce
1 teaspoon pepper
1–2 teaspoons dried chilli flakes
175 g (6 oz) dried white rice noodles, soaked and drained
coriander leaves and lime quarters, to garnish

1 Heat the stock in a saucepan and add all the ingredients, except the noodles.

2 Bring to the boil for 30 seconds, then lower the heat and simmer for 5 minutes.

3 Add the noodles and simmer for a further 2 minutes.

4 Pour the soup into warmed serving bowls and garnish with coriander leaves and lime quarters.

Apple and walnut salad

alcohol free ✓ | citrus free ✗ | dairy free ✓ | gluten free ✓ | wheat free ✓

Serves 6
Preparation time: 15–20 minutes

Per serving
Energy 70 kcals/296 kJ | Protein 2 g | Carbohydrate 5 g | Fat 5 g
Fibre 2 g

1 iceberg lettuce, sliced
2 bunches of watercress, chopped
1 apple, peeled, cubed and tossed in lemon juice
25 g (1 oz) walnuts, chopped
1 tablespoon walnut oil
2 tablespoons wine vinegar
salt and pepper

1 Mix the lettuce with the watercress and apple in a serving bowl.

2 Sprinkle the walnuts over the salad and drizzle over the oil and
vinegar. Season to taste with salt and pepper and toss the salad
well just before serving.

Variation
The partnership of apples and walnuts is delicious, but other fruit and
nut combinations can work equally well. Try peach and hazelnuts
with hazelnut oil, for example, or apricots and almonds.

Provençal pasta salad

alcohol free ✓ | citrus free ✕ | dairy free ✕ | gluten free ✕ | wheat free ✕

Serves 6
Preparation time: 20 minutes, plus cooling
Cooking time: about 10–12 minutes

Per serving
Energy 240 kcals/1009 kJ | Protein 15 g | Carbohydrate 27 g | Fat 9 g
Fibre 4 g

175 g (6 oz) rigatoni or penne
4 tablespoons low-fat mayonnaise
2 tablespoons lemon juice
6 tomatoes, skinned, deseeded and chopped
125 g (4 oz) French beans, cooked
12 black olives, pitted
200 g (7 oz) can tuna in brine, drained and flaked
salt and pepper
1 small lettuce, shredded, to serve
50 g (2 oz) can anchovy fillets, drained and washed, to garnish

1 Cook the pasta in a large saucepan of lightly salted water for 10–12 minutes, or according to the packet instructions, until tender. Rinse under cold running water, then drain well and leave to cool.

2 Turn the pasta into a bowl and mix with the mayonnaise, lemon juice, tomatoes, beans, olives and flaked tuna. Season to taste with salt and pepper. Serve on a bed of shredded lettuce and garnish with anchovies.

Vegetable dishes

Tagliatelle sicilienne

alcohol free ✓ | citrus free ✓ | dairy free ✓ | gluten free ✗ | wheat free ✗

Serves 4
Preparation time: 10 minutes
Cooking time: 20–27 minutes

Per serving
Energy 370 kcals/1490 kJ | Protein 14 g | Carbohydrate 68 g | Fat 5 g
Fibre 3 g

1 tablespoon olive oil
2 onions, chopped
2 garlic cloves, chopped
1 large aubergine, diced
400 g (13 oz) can chopped plum tomatoes
2 teaspoons chopped basil
375 g (12 oz) fresh tagliatelle
salt and pepper

1 Heat the oil in a saucepan and fry the onion, garlic and aubergine
for 2–3 minutes. Add the tomatoes and their juice, together with
the basil, and season to taste with salt and pepper. Simmer for
15–20 minutes.

2 Cook the pasta in a large saucepan of lightly salted boiling water
for 3–4 minutes until tender.

3 Drain the pasta, turn it into a warmed serving dish and top with
the aubergine mixture.

Yellow rice with mushrooms

alcohol free ✓ | citrus free ✓ | dairy free ✓ | gluten free ✕ | wheat free ✕

Serves 4
Preparation time: 10 minutes
Cooking time: 3–4 minutes

Per serving
Energy 226 kcals/952 kJ | Protein 6 g | Carbohydrate 42 g | Fat 5 g
Fibre 3 g

1 tablespoon groundnut oil
500 g (1 lb) cold cooked rice
125 g (4 oz) mangetout, topped and tailed
125 g (4 oz) button mushrooms, halved
125 g (4 oz) bamboo shoots
1 teaspoon turmeric
2 teaspoons sugar
1 tablespoon Tamari (wheat-free soy sauce)
1 teaspoon salt
pepper

To Garnish:
1 tablespoon sliced garlic, deep-fried until crispy
1 large red chilli, deseeded and cut into strips

1 Heat the oil in a wok or large frying pan. Add the rice, stir well, then add the remaining ingredients. Stir-fry over a low heat until thoroughly combined. Increase the heat and stir for a further 1–2 minutes, making sure that the rice does not stick to the pan.

2 Turn on to a serving dish, garnish with the crispy garlic and chilli and serve immediately.

Root vegetable bake

alcohol free ✓ | citrus free ✓ | dairy free ✗ | gluten free ✓ | wheat free ✓

Serves 4
Preparation time: 20 minutes
Cooking time: 40–50 minutes

Per serving
Energy 218 kcals/920 kJ | Protein 8 g | Carbohydrate 38 g | Fat 5 g
Fibre 8 g

500 g (1 lb) new potatoes
250 g (8 oz) swede, cubed
300 g (10 oz) parsnips, sliced
250 g (8 oz) carrots, cut into matchsticks
65 ml (2½ fl oz) vegetable stock
50 g (2 oz) Edam cheese, grated
salt and pepper

To Garnish:
tomato slices
1 tablespoon chopped parsley

1 Cook the potatoes in a saucepan of boiling salted water until just
tender. Cut into 5 mm (¼ inch) slices. Cook the remaining
vegetables together in a large saucepan of boiling salted water
until just tender. Drain all the vegetables and place in layers in a
deep ovenproof dish, finishing with a border of overlapping
potato slices. Pour over the stock, sprinkle with the cheese and
season to taste with pepper.

2 Bake in a preheated oven at 180°C (350°F), Gas Mark 4, for
15–20 minutes until the cheese has melted and the vegetables are
heated through. Serve garnished with tomato slices and parsley.

Caponata

alcohol free ✓ | citrus free ✓ | dairy free ✓ | gluten free ✓ | wheat free ✓

Serves 6
Preparation time: 35 minutes
Cooking time: 1¼ hours

Per serving
Energy 123 kcals/512 kJ | Protein 4 g | Carbohydrate 8 g | Fat 9 g
Fibre 4 g

2 tablespoons olive oil
1 onion, thinly sliced
2 celery sticks, diced
3 aubergines, cut into 1.5 cm (½ inch) dice
150 ml (¼ pint) passata
3 tablespoons wine vinegar
1 yellow pepper, cored, deseeded and finely sliced
1 red pepper, cored, deseeded and finely sliced
25 g (1 oz) anchovy fillets, soaked in warm water, drained and dried
50 g (2 oz) capers, roughly chopped
25 g (1 oz) black olives, pitted and sliced
25 g (1 oz) green olives, pitted and sliced
25 g (1 oz) pine nuts
2 tablespoons chopped parsley, to garnish

1 Heat the oil in a saucepan and fry the onion until soft and golden. Add the celery and cook for 2–3 minutes. Add the aubergine and cook gently for 3 minutes, stirring occasionally.

2 Add the passata and cook gently until it has been absorbed. Spoon in the vinegar and cook for 1 minute. Add the peppers, anchovies, capers, olives and pine nuts, and cook for a further 3 minutes.

3 Transfer the mixture to an ovenproof dish and bake, covered, in a preheated oven at 180°C (350°F), Gas Mark 4, for about 1 hour. Serve lukewarm or cold, sprinkled with chopped parsley.

Scalloped potatoes

alcohol free ✓ | citrus free ✓ | dairy free ✗ | gluten free ✓ | wheat free ✓

Serves 6
Preparation time: 20 minutes, plus standing
Cooking time: 1 hour 20 minutes

Per serving
Energy 203 kcals/853 kJ | Protein 5 g | Carbohydrate 31 g | Fat 7 g
Fibre 2 g

2 teaspoons vegetable oil
75 ml (3 fl oz) low-fat soured cream
350 ml (12 fl oz) skimmed milk
25 g (1 oz) butter or margarine
1 tablespoon cornflour
750 g (1½ lb) potatoes, cut into 5 mm (¼ inch) slices
½ onion, diced
pepper

To Garnish:
paprika
thyme sprigs

1 Brush a casserole or ovenproof dish with oil. Whisk together the soured cream, milk, butter or margarine and cornflour, and season to taste with pepper.

2 Line the dish with one-third of the potato slices. Pour one-third of the soured cream mixture over the potatoes. Sprinkle half of the onion over the soured cream mixture. Repeat the layers in order: one-third of the potatoes, one-third of the soured cream mixture and the remaining onion. Arrange the remaining potatoes on the top and pour the remaining soured cream mixture over the top of the potatoes. Cover with foil and bake in a preheated oven at 180°C (350°F), Gas Mark 4, for 1 hour. Remove the foil and bake for a further 20 minutes.

3 Sprinkle with paprika and thyme sprigs, then allow to stand for 5 minutes before serving.

Green pea stew with saffron and mint

alcohol free ✓ | citrus free ✓ | dairy free ✕ | gluten free ✕ | wheat free ✕

Serves 4
Preparation time: 20 minutes, plus standing
Cooking time: 30–40 minutes

Per serving
Energy 420 kcals/1754 kJ | Protein 16 g | Carbohydrate 25 g | Fat 29 g
Fibre 10 g

pinch of saffron threads
300 ml (½ pint) boiling water
50 g (2 oz) butter
3 shallots or 1 small onion, finely chopped
1 garlic clove, crushed
75 g (3 oz) pancetta or streaky bacon, cut into strips (optional)
500 g (1 lb) shelled peas, thawed if frozen
2 little gem lettuces, cut into wide strips
1–2 teaspoons caster sugar
2 egg yolks, beaten
2 tablespoons chopped mint
salt and pepper

Topping:
25 g (1 oz) butter
75 g (3 oz) fresh white breadcrumbs
25 g (1 oz) Parmesan or Pecorino cheese, finely grated

1 Put the saffron into a small bowl and pour over the boiling water. Leave to infuse for 10 minutes.

2 Melt the butter in a large flameproof casserole and fry the shallots or onion and garlic for 5–6 minutes until soft but not coloured. Add the pancetta or bacon, if using, and cook for a further 1–2 minutes. Add the peas, lettuce, 1 teaspoon of caster sugar and the saffron and its water. Cover the casserole and cook for 10–15 minutes until the peas are tender. If using frozen peas, add to the pan after 5 minutes. Season to taste with salt and pepper, and add more sugar, if necessary.

3 Meanwhile, to make the breadcrumb topping, melt the butter in a frying pan and fry the breadcrumbs, stirring frequently, until golden brown. Remove from the heat, leave to cool slightly, then stir in the grated cheese.

4 Beat the egg yolks in a small bowl and, when the peas are cooked, ladle out a little of liquid from the casserole and stir into the egg yolks. When the mixture is well combined, pour it back into the casserole and stir until the sauce has thickened. Do not allow it to boil or it will curdle. Stir in the mint and serve sprinkled with the breadcrumb topping.

Noodles with chinese vegetables

alcohol free ✓ | citrus free ✓ | dairy free ✓ | gluten free × | wheat free ×

Serves 4
Preparation time: 15 minutes
Cooking time: 8–10 minutes

Per serving
Energy 337 kcals/1419 kJ | Protein 10 g | Carbohydrate 50 g | Fat 12 g
Fibre 4 g

250 g (8 oz) dried egg noodles
2 tablespoons groundnut oil
50 g (2 oz) leek, sliced
25 g (1 oz) oyster mushrooms, torn
1 celery stick and leaf, chopped
125 g (4 oz) Chinese leaves, sliced
25 g (1 oz) cauliflower florets
2 tablespoons soy sauce
1½ teaspoons sugar
½ teaspoon salt
1 teaspoon pepper
2 tablespoons sliced garlic, deep-fried until crispy
coriander leaves, to garnish

1 Cook the noodles in a large saucepan of boiling water for 5–6 minutes, or according to the packet instructions, until just tender. Drain and rinse under cold running water to prevent further cooking.

2 Heat the oil in a wok or large frying pan over a moderate heat, then add all the remaining ingredients one by one, including the noodles, stirring after each addition.

3 Stir-fry for 3–4 minutes, adding more oil, if necessary. Check and adjust the seasoning, if necessary. Serve immediately, garnished with coriander leaves.

Dhal

alcohol free ✓ | citrus free ✓ | dairy free ✓ | gluten free ✓ | wheat free ✓

Serves 4
Preparation time: about 15 minutes, plus soaking
Cooking time: 55 minutes

Per serving
Energy 256 kcals/1083 kJ | Protein 17 g | Carbohydrate 37 g | Fat 6 g
Fibre 2 g

250 g (8 oz) dried green lentils, soaked in cold water overnight
1 medium onion, finely chopped
2.5 cm (1 inch) piece of fresh root ginger, bruised
2 bay leaves, crushed
2 green chillies, chopped
1 tablespoon chopped fresh coriander
5 teaspoons olive oil
2 large garlic cloves, crushed
1 teaspoon ground coriander
½ teaspoon ground cumin
½ teaspoon garam masala
375 g (12 oz) tomatoes, skinned, deseeded and chopped
salt

1 Drain the lentils and put them into a pan with the onion, ginger, bay leaves, chillies, fresh coriander, 2 teaspoons of the oil and sufficient water just to cover. Bring to the boil, then lower the heat and simmer for about 45 minutes until the lentils are just tender. If the lentils become too dry, simply add a little extra liquid to the pan.

2 Heat the remaining oil and fry the garlic for 2–3 minutes. Add the ground coriander, cumin and garam masala, and fry for a further minute. Add the tomatoes and salt to taste, and heat through.

3 Stir the tomato and spice mixture into the lentils. Heat through gently for about 5 minutes and serve piping hot.

Fabulous fish

Smoked salmon and asparagus fettuccine

alcohol free ✓ | citrus free ✓ | dairy free ✕ | gluten free ✕ | wheat free ✕

Serves 4
Preparation time: 10 minutes
Cooking time: 15–20 minutes

Per serving
Energy 686 kcals/2783 kJ | Protein 22 g | Carbohydrate 60 g | Fat 40 g
Fibre 1 g

175 g (6 oz) asparagus tips
375 g (12 oz) fresh fettuccine or tagliatelle
125 g (4 oz) smoked salmon, cut into thin strips
300 ml (½ pint) double cream
1 tablespoon tarragon leaves
salt and pepper
Parmesan cheese shavings, to garnish

1 Blanch the asparagus tips in boiling salted water for 3–5 minutes. Drain in a colander and refresh under cold running water. Drain thoroughly and pat dry.

2 Cook the pasta in a large saucepan of lightly salted boiling water for 8–10 minutes, or according to the packet instructions, until tender. Drain and return to the pan. Toss over a low heat with the asparagus, smoked salmon, cream, tarragon and salt and pepper to taste until heated through.

3 Transfer to a warmed serving dish and garnish with wafer-thin shavings of Parmesan.

Grilled salmon with potato cakes and watercress sauce

alcohol free ✓ | citrus free ✗ | dairy free ✗ | gluten free ✓ | wheat free ✓

Serves 4
Preparation time: 20 minutes
Cooking time: 15–20 minutes

Per serving
Energy 536 kcals/2227 kJ | Protein 28 g | Carbohydrate 22 g | Fat 38 g
Fibre 2 g

425 g (14 oz) grated raw potato
3–4 tablespoons olive oil
4 salmon fillets, about 125 g (4 oz) each
25 g (1 oz) butter

Watercress Sauce:
2–3 bunches of watercress
250 ml (8 fl oz) crème fraîche
lemon juice, to taste
salt and pepper

1 To make the watercress sauce, chop the watercress, reserving 4 sprigs for garnish, then put it into a saucepan with the crème fraîche and stir together. Add lemon juice and salt and pepper to taste, and set aside.

2 Put the grated potato into a bowl and season to taste with salt and pepper. Divide the mixture into 4 cakes. Heat the oil in a frying pan and fry the potato cakes over a moderate heat until browned all over and soft inside. Remove from the pan and set aside to keep warm.

3 Meanwhile, season the salmon fillets with salt and pepper. Line the grill pan with a piece of greased foil and arrange the fillets on top. Dot with butter and cook under a preheated grill for 4–5 minutes on each side until cooked through.

4 Heat the watercress sauce gently – it may be served hot or cold.

5 To serve, place a potato cake on each plate, put a salmon fillet on top and pour the sauce over. Garnish with watercress sprigs and serve immediately.

Baked herrings with ginger and honey sauce

alcohol free ✕ | citrus free ✓ | dairy free ✓ | gluten free ✓ | wheat free ✓

Serves 4
Preparation time: 20 minutes, plus marinating
Cooking time: 25–30 minutes

Per serving
Energy 415 kcals/1733 kJ | Protein 22 g | Carbohydrate 31 g | Fat 23 g
Fibre 3 g

4 herrings, filleted
2 carrots, cut into matchsticks
2 celery sticks, cut into matchsticks
1 red pepper, cored, deseeded and thinly sliced
1 green pepper, cored, deseeded and thinly sliced
1 large onion, thinly sliced

Ginger and Honey Sauce:
2 tablespoons red wine vinegar
1 tablespoon Tamari (wheat-free soy sauce)
2 tablespoons dry sherry
2 tablespoons clear honey
3 tablespoons water
1 teaspoon ground ginger
2 tablespoons cornflour
pinch of cayenne pepper
2.5 cm (1 inch) piece of fresh root ginger, peeled and finely chopped
pepper

1 To make the sauce, put all the ingredients into a small jug and stir well.

2 Put the fish into a shallow baking dish and pour over the sauce. Cover and leave to marinate in the refrigerator for at least 2 hours.

3 Turn the fish in the sauce and add the carrots, celery, peppers and onion. Cover the dish with foil and bake in a preheated oven at 190°C (375°F), Gas Mark 5, for 25–30 minutes.

4 Divide the vegetables among 4 warmed plates, arrange the herrings on top and serve immediately.

Red mullet with fennel and rouille

alcohol free ✓ | citrus free ✗ | dairy free ✓ | gluten free ✓ | wheat free ✓

Serves 6
Preparation time: 25 minutes
Cooking time: 20 minutes

Per serving
Energy 454 kcals/1886 kJ | Protein 30 g | Carbohydrate 1 g | Fat 37 g
Fibre 0 g

6 red mullet, filleted
2 small fennel bulbs
2 tablespoons olive oil
sea salt and pepper

Rouille:
3 garlic cloves, peeled
1–2 red chillies, deseeded and coarsely chopped
2 egg yolks
175–250 ml (6–8 fl oz) olive oil
lemon juice (optional)

To Serve:
steamed green beans
lightly roasted tomatoes

1 Rinse the red mullet fillets and pat dry. Slice the fennel bulbs very thinly. Brush the fish with a little oil, then wrap the fillets around slices of fennel. Put them on to a baking sheet lined with greased foil and bake in a preheated oven at 180°C (350°F), Gas Mark 4, for 20 minutes until cooked.

2 To make the rouille, pound the garlic very thoroughly using a pestle and mortar. Add the chopped chillies and pound to a paste. Whisk the egg yolks in a large bowl. Whisk in the garlic paste, mixing very well.

3 Add a few drops of oil, beating thoroughly, then a few more once the first has been absorbed. Keep on adding the oil, a little at a time, beating constantly and adding more oil only when the previous addition has been amalgamated. The mixture will be very thick. Season lightly with salt, generously with pepper and add a few drops of lemon juice, if liked. This is not traditional but gives a fresher flavour.

4 Serve the mullet immediately on a bed of green beans and tomatoes, with the rouille offered separately.

Swordfish casserole

alcohol free ✓ | citrus free ✓ | dairy free ✓ | gluten free ✓ | wheat free ✓

Serves 4
Preparation time: 20 minutes
Cooking time: 45–55 minutes

Per serving
Energy 507 kcals/2140 kJ | Protein 40 g | Carbohydrate 62 g | Fat 13 g
Fibre 4 g

1 tablespoon olive oil
2 red peppers, cored, deseeded and chopped
1 onion, chopped
1 garlic clove, finely chopped
1 tablespoon white wine vinegar
1 tablespoon tomato purée
1 tablespoon finely chopped thyme, plus extra to garnish
250 ml (8 fl oz) fish stock
250 g (8 oz) celery, sliced
750 g (1½ lb) swordfish, cubed
250 g (8 oz) long-grain rice
300 ml (½ pint) water
8 pitted black olives, sliced
salt and pepper

1 Heat the olive oil in a frying pan and fry the peppers and onions gently until just soft. Add the garlic, vinegar, tomato purée, thyme and stock. Simmer for 5 minutes, then season to taste with salt and pepper.

2 Turn the mixture into a food processor or blender and blend until smooth, or push with a wooden spoon through a fine sieve. Transfer the purée to a flameproof casserole. Add the celery and swordfish and bring to the boil. Cover and bake in a preheated oven at 180°C (350°F), Gas Mark 4, for 20–30 minutes.

3 Meanwhile, put the rice into a saucepan, add the water, season to taste with salt and bring to the boil. Lower the heat, cover and simmer for 12–14 minutes until the rice is tender and all the liquid has been absorbed.

4 Remove the rice from the heat, fluff up with a fork, stir in the olives and keep warm. Transfer the fish to a warmed serving dish with the rice and serve, garnished with thyme.

Madras fish kebabs

alcohol free ✓ | citrus free ✗ | dairy free ✗ | gluten free ✓ | wheat free ✓

Serves 4
Preparation time: 20 minutes, plus marinating
Cooking time: about 6 minutes

Per serving
Energy 153 kcals/648 kJ | Protein 31 g | Carbohydrate 4 g | Fat 2 g
Fibre 0 g

4 tablespoons natural yogurt
3 tablespoons lime juice
1 garlic clove, crushed
1 teaspoon curry powder
6 drops Tabasco sauce
1 thin slice of fresh root ginger, finely chopped
500 g (1 lb) monkfish or other firm white fish,
    cut into 2.5 cm (1 inch) cubes
12 raw tiger prawns, peeled and deveined
12 mussels, cooked and shelled
salt and pepper

To Garnish:
1 tablespoon roughly chopped coriander
lime wedges

1 Mix the yogurt with the lime juice, garlic, curry powder, Tabasco, ginger and salt and pepper to taste.

2 Stir the fish, prawns and mussels lightly into the spiced yogurt mixture, cover and chill for 4 hours.

3 Thread the pieces of fish, prawns and mussels alternately on to 4 metal skewers. Brush off any excess yogurt marinade and reserve.

4 Put the kebabs on to a lightly greased baking sheet and cook under a preheated hot grill for about 6 minutes until the fish is just tender, brushing occasionally with yogurt marinade. Arrange the kebabs on a platter, sprinkle with coriander and garnish with lime wedges.

Monkfish in creamy tomato sauce

alcohol free ✕ | citrus free ✓ | dairy free ✕ | gluten free ✕ | wheat free ✕

Serves 4
Preparation time: 15 minutes
Cooking time: about 20 minutes

Per serving
Energy 530 kcals/2206 kJ | Protein 23 g | Carbohydrate 14 g | Fat 38 g
Fibre 2 g

500 g (1 lb) monkfish, cut into 4 cm (1½ inch) pieces
50 g (2 oz) plain flour
2 tablespoons sunflower oil
50 g (2 oz) butter
300 ml (10 fl oz) white wine
6 small tomatoes, skinned, deseeded and cut into quarters
175 ml (6 fl oz) double cream
3 tablespoons snipped chives
salt and pepper

1 Coat the fish pieces with the flour and season to taste with salt
and pepper. Heat the oil with the butter in a saucepan and fry the
fish gently for 4–6 minutes until cooked. Remove from the pan
and keep warm.

2 Pour any excess oil out of the pan. Add the wine and boil rapidly
until reduced by half. Add the tomatoes, cream and chives and
boil for 2 minutes. Season to taste, stir in the monkfish and serve
immediately.

Prawn and mango curry

alcohol free ✓ | citrus free ✗ | dairy free ✓ | gluten free ✓ | wheat free ✓

Serves 4
Preparation time: 20 minutes
Cooking time: about 15 minutes

Per serving
Energy 230 kcals/966 kJ | Protein 4 g | Carbohydrate 15 g | Fat 13 g
Fibre 2 g

2 tablespoons groundnut oil
1 red onion, finely chopped
2 garlic cloves, crushed
4 tablespoons mild curry paste
400 ml (14 fl oz) coconut milk
4 tablespoons lemon juice
2 tablespoons ground almonds
24 raw tiger prawns, peeled and deveined
1 small ripe mango, peeled and diced
salt

1 Heat the oil in a heavy-based saucepan and fry the onion and
garlic gently, stirring frequently, for about 4 minutes or until soft.
Stir in the curry paste and cook for a further 2 minutes.

2 Add the coconut milk and lemon juice to the pan, stir to mix and
simmer for 3 minutes. Add the ground almonds, prawns and salt
to taste, then simmer gently for a further 3 minutes until the
prawns have turned pink and the sauce has thickened slightly.

3 Stir the mango into the curry and heat through for 1 minute.
Taste and adjust the seasoning, if necessary. Transfer the curry to
a warmed serving dish and serve.

Meat meals

Andalusian chicken

alcohol free ✓ | citrus free ✗ | dairy free ✓ | gluten free ✓ | wheat free ✓

Serves 8
Preparation time: 30 minutes
Cooking time: 1¾ hours

Per serving
Energy 350 kcals/1479 kJ | Protein 29 g | Carbohydrate 47 g | Fat 7 g
Fibre 4 g

1.75 kg (3½ lb) roasting chicken
1 teaspoon dried mixed herbs
1 teaspoon vegetable oil
250 g (8 oz) Spanish onions, chopped
500 g (1 lb) green peppers, cored, deseeded and diced
4 tomatoes, skinned, deseeded and roughly chopped
2 garlic cloves, crushed
250 g (8 oz) peas, cooked
375 g (12 oz) long-grain rice
900 ml (1½ pints) chicken stock
pinch of powdered saffron
1 bay leaf
salt and pepper

To Garnish:
lemon slices
chopped parsley

1 Sprinkle the chicken with salt and pepper to taste and the herbs, then stand it in a roasting tin. Pour a cup of water round the chicken. Cover loosely with greased greaseproof paper or foil and roast in a preheated oven at 200°C (400°F), Gas Mark 6, for 1½ hours. Leave the chicken to cool slightly, then discard the skin, strip the flesh from the bones and cut it into bite-sized pieces. Set aside. Use the chicken carcass and giblets to make chicken stock, in which to cook the rice.

2 Heat the oil in a large saucepan and fry the onions, peppers, tomatoes and garlic gently until soft and golden. Stir in the cooked peas.

3 Meanwhile, cook the rice in the chicken stock in a saucepan with the saffron and bay leaf for about 10 minutes until the rice is tender. Drain, if necessary (the rice should be quite dry), and remove the bay leaf.

4 Stir the chicken and rice into the onion and pepper mixture. Pile into a large, warmed serving dish and garnish with lemon slices and parsley.

Stir-fried chicken with crunchy vegetables

alcohol free ✓ | citrus free ✓ | dairy free ✓ | gluten free ✓ | wheat free ✓

Serves 4
Preparation time: 20 minutes
Cooking time: 6–10 minutes

Per serving
Energy 204 kcals/859 kJ | Protein 31 g | Carbohydrate 9 g | Fat 5 g
Fibre 3 g

1 teaspoon vegetable oil
500 g (1 lb) skinless, boneless chicken breast, cut into thin strips
   across the grain
125 g (4 oz) white cabbage, finely shredded
125 g (4 oz) bean sprouts
1 large green pepper, cored, deseeded and cut into thin strips
2 medium carrots, cut into strips
2 garlic cloves, crushed
pepper

Sauce:
2 teaspoons cornflour
4 tablespoons water
3 tablespoons Tamari (wheat-free soy sauce)

1 To prepare the sauce, mix the cornflour to a thin paste with the water, then stir in the soy sauce and set aside.

2 Heat a wok or large frying pan until hot. Add the oil and heat until hot. Stir-fry the chicken strips quickly for 3–4 minutes until lightly coloured on all sides.

3 Remove the pan from the heat and transfer the chicken to a plate with a slotted spoon. Set aside.

4 Return the pan to a moderate heat until hot and stir-fry all the vegetables and garlic for 2–3 minutes until the green pepper is just beginning to soften.

5 Stir the sauce to combine, then pour into the pan. Increase the heat to high and toss the ingredients until the sauce thickens and coats the vegetables. Add the chicken with its juices and toss for 1–2 minutes until all the ingredients are combined. Add pepper to taste and serve immediately.

Chicken en cocotte

alcohol free ✗ | citrus free ✓ | dairy free ✓ | gluten free ✓ | wheat free ✓

Serves 6
Preparation time: 20 minutes
Cooking time: 50 minutes

Per serving
Energy 224 kcals/940 kJ | Protein 25 g | Carbohydrate 8 g | Fat 6 g
Fibre 3 g

1.5 kg (3 lb) chicken, skinned and jointed
1 teaspoon vegetable oil
25 g (1 oz) lean smoked ham, diced
4 small onions, chopped
1 garlic clove, crushed
2 tablespoons brandy
6 tomatoes, peeled and chopped
3 carrots, chopped
2 celery sticks, cut into 4 cm (1½ inch) lengths
½ teaspoon chopped thyme
1 bay leaf
300 ml (½ pint) red wine
salt and pepper
chopped parsley, to garnish

1 Season the chicken portions with salt and pepper. Heat the oil in a flameproof casserole and add the diced ham and chicken portions. Cook until golden on all sides. Take out the meats and set aside.

2 Fry the onions and garlic in the pan until softened, stirring. Return the chicken and ham to the pan. Pour on the brandy and flambé the meat very carefully. Now add the tomatoes, carrots, celery, thyme, bay leaf and red wine. Bring to the boil, cover and simmer for about 30 minutes, until the chicken and vegetables are tender. Remove the bay leaf before serving and sprinkle with chopped parsley. Serve immediately.

Catalan pork stew

alcohol free ✓ | citrus free ✓ | dairy free ✓ | gluten free ✓ | wheat free ✓

Serves 4
Preparation time: 20 minutes
Cooking time: 1¼ hours

Per serving
Energy 424 kcals/1769 kJ | Protein 41 g | Carbohydrate 9 g | Fat 25 g
Fibre 2 g

4 tablespoons olive oil
750 g (1½ lb) lean pork, cut into 2.5 cm (1 inch) cubes
1 large onion, sliced
2 garlic cloves, crushed
400 g (13 oz) can chopped tomatoes
1 green pepper, cored, deseeded and chopped
1½ teaspoons paprika
150 ml (¼ pint) chicken stock
salt and pepper
1 tablespoon chopped coriander, to garnish
rice, to serve

1 Heat the oil in a large heavy-based pan and fry the pork gently, turning occasionally, until golden brown all over. Remove from the pan with a slotted spoon and set aside.

2 Add the onion and garlic to the cooking juices in the pan and cook until soft and golden. Return the meat to the pan and stir in the tomatoes, green pepper, paprika and stock. Season to taste with salt and pepper. Bring to the boil, cover tightly and simmer gently for about 1 hour until the meat is tender.

3 Serve the pork, garnished with coriander, with plain boiled rice.

Stir-fried liver and spinach with ginger

alcohol free ✗ | citrus free ✓ | dairy free ✓ | gluten free ✓ | wheat free ✓

Serves 4
Preparation time: 10 minutes
Cooking time: 4–5 minutes

Per serving
Energy 306 kcals/1278 kJ | Protein 23 g | Carbohydrate 14 g | Fat 18 g
Fibre 5 g

375 g (12 oz) lamb's liver, cut into thin slices
2 tablespoons cornflour
4 tablespoons sunflower oil
500 g (1 lb) spinach leaves
1 teaspoon salt
2 thin slices of fresh root ginger, chopped
1 tablespoon Tamari (wheat-free soy sauce)
1 tablespoon Chinese rice wine or dry sherry
finely chopped spring onions, to garnish

1 Blanch the slices of liver in boiling water for a few seconds. Drain, then coat with cornflour.

2 Heat 2 tablespoons of the oil in a wok or large frying pan and stir-fry the spinach with the salt for 2 minutes. Remove from the pan and arrange around the edge of a warmed serving dish. Keep warm.

3 Wipe the pan clean with kitchen paper. Heat the remaining oil in the pan until very hot and stir-fry the ginger, liver, Tamari and wine or sherry quickly for 1–2 minutes – avoid overcooking or the liver will become tough. Pour the mixture over the spinach and garnish with spring onions.

Lamb with couscous

alcohol free ✓ | citrus free ✓ | dairy free ✕ | gluten free ✕ | wheat free ✕

Serves 4
Preparation time: 30 minutes
Cooking time: 1 hour

Per serving
Energy 703 kcals/2936 kJ | Protein 41 g | Carbohydrate 91 g | Fat 22 g
Fibre 6 g

500 g (1 lb) lean boneless lamb, cut into large cubes
900 ml (1½ pints) water
2 onions, quartered and thickly sliced
2 garlic cloves, crushed
pinch of saffron threads, crushed
1 teaspoon ground cinnamon
½ teaspoon paprika
1 red chilli, deseeded and finely chopped
½ teaspoon ground ginger
500 g (1 lb) couscous
250 g (8 oz) small carrots, quartered lengthways
250 g (8 oz) small turnips, quartered
250 g (8 oz) kohlrabi or celeriac, cut into large chunks
250 g (8 oz) courgettes, quartered lengthways
250 g (8 oz) broad beans
4 tomatoes, quartered
large bunch of coriander, chopped
large bunch of flat leaf parsley, chopped
40 g (1½ oz) unsalted butter
salt and pepper

1 Put the lamb into a large heavy-based pan. Add the water, the onions, garlic, saffron, cinnamon, paprika, chilli, ginger and salt and pepper to taste. Bring to the boil, remove any scum from the surface, cover and simmer very gently for about 30 minutes.

2 Meanwhile, soak the couscous in a bowl of cold water for 10–15 minutes then stir gently with a wooden spoon to break up any lumps. Drain in a colander. Line a steamer with some muslin and tip in the couscous.

3 Add the carrots, turnips and kholrabi or celeriac to the lamb. Put the steamer containing the couscous over the pan with the lamb (it should not touch the stew below) and steam gently for 10 minutes.

4 Add the courgettes, broad beans, tomatoes, coriander and parsley to the lamb and cook for a further 5–10 minutes or until the vegetables, lamb and couscous are tender.

5 Fork through the couscous to separate the grains, then turn on to a large serving plate. Dot the butter over the top, stir it in and season with salt and pepper. Form into a mound with a large well in the centre and place the lamb in the well using a slotted spoon. Lift the vegetables from the cooking broth and place on and around the lamb. Serve the broth in a separate bowl.

Stir-fried beef with peppers

alcohol free ✗ | citrus free ✓ | dairy free ✓ | gluten free ✓ | wheat free ✓

Serves 6
Preparation time: 20 minutes
Cooking time: 10–12 minutes

Per serving
Energy 160 kcals/667 kJ | Protein 19 g | Carbohydrate 4 g | Fat 7 g
Fibre 1 g

1 tablespoon olive oil
1 onion, finely sliced
1 large garlic clove, cut into thin strips
500 g (1 lb) fillet steak, cut into thin strips
1 red pepper, cored, deseeded and cut into matchsticks
1 green pepper, cored, deseeded and cut into matchsticks
1 tablespoon Tamari (wheat-free soy sauce)
2 tablespoons dry sherry
1 tablespoon chopped rosemary
salt and pepper
rice, to serve

1 Heat the oil in a wok or large frying pan and stir-fry the onion and garlic for 2 minutes.

2 Add the strips of beef and stir-fry quickly until evenly browned on all sides and almost tender.

3 Add the strips of pepper and stir-fry for a further 2 minutes.

4 Add the Tamari, sherry, salt and pepper to taste and the rosemary, and stir-fry for a further 1–2 minutes. Serve immediately with rice.

Glossary

ALLERGEN A normally harmless substance or food that in someone who has a tendency to allergy provokes an allergic reaction.

ATOPY A tendency to allergy.

CORTICOSTEROIDS A group of drugs similar to the corticosteroid hormones produced by the cortex of the adrenal glands with anti-inflammatory properties.

DERMIS The thicker inner layer of the skin.

EMOLLIENT A substance that soothes and softens the skin used in creams, ointments and lotions.

EPIDERMIS The thin outer layer of the skin.

ERYTHEMA Acute inflammation of the skin causing redness.

HOMEOSTASIS The body's internal balance.

IMMUNOGLOBULIN A type of protein produced by the immune system also known as an antibody.

IMMUNOSUPPRESSIVE DRUGS A group of drugs that reduce the activity of the immune system.

KERATIN A hard fibrous protein found in the epidermis as well as in nails and hair.

KERATINOCYTES Skin cells that manufacture keratin.

LANGERHANS CELLS Specialized cells which are produced in the bone marrow and form part of the body's immune response which protects against disease and infection.

LICHENIFICATION Thickening and hardening of the skin caused by repeated scratching.

MAST CELLS A type of cell found in body tissues that releases histamine, a chemical that produces the symptoms of allergy.

MELANIN The brown pigment found in the epidermis which absorbs ultraviolet light and protects us from sun damage.

MELANOCYTES A group of spider-shaped skin cells that manufacture melanin.

MERKEL CELLS A type of cell found in the epidermis that helps us to sense touch.

METABOLIC PROCESSES Chemical processes that take place in the body.

PROSTAGLANDINS A group of chemicals made by the body that work in a similar way to hormones.

SEBUM An oily secretion produced by the sebaceous glands which are found in the skin.

SENSITIZATION The initial exposure to an allergen or other substance which leads to an immune reaction.

URTICARIA Itchy raised weals surrounded by areas of red inflammation. Also known as nettle rash or hives.

General Index

A

absorbency 13
ACE vitamins 102
acid mantle 13
acids, fruit 50
acne 19, 21
acupuncture 81–3
adaptogens 88
additives 48, 109
adrenal glands 68
adrenaline 36, 56
adults 32, 69, 107
age factors 25, 32
AHAs see Alpha
  Hydroxy Acids
alcohol 27, 109
allergens
  see also house dust
    mites: triggers
  chromate 38
  eczema causes 26
  hair dyes 38
Immunoglobulin E
  27–8
keratinocytes 14
lanolin 38
metals 38
perfumes 38
pets 55–6, 58
plants 38, 53
pollen 53, 58
preservatives 38
rubber 38
allergic contact
  dermatitis 37–8
allergic reactions 27–8
  anti-histamines 71
  Chinese herbalism 87
  exclusion diets 112
  genetic factors 24
  immediate food
    hypersensitivity 105
  tests 109–14
Alpha Hydroxy Acids
(AHAs) 50
ammonia 18
anabolic steroids 67
anaphylactic shock 36
animal dander 30, 55,
  109
anti-bacterial
  substances 40
anti-histamines 40, 59,
  70–2, 120
antibiotics 70
antibodies 28, 105
antioxidants 102, 120
antiseptics 70
aqueous cream 49
asanas, hatha yoga 97
aspirin 84
asteatotic eczema 14,
  25, 41
asthma 25, 27, 29, 35,
  53, 55
Atherton, David 86

atopic eczema 30–6
  adults 32
  allergic reactions 27
  causes 26–8
  children 25, 30–1, 60
  delayed food hypersensitivity 107
  food sensitivity 100, 107
  food supplements 113
  immunosuppressive drugs 74
  itchiness 31–3
  medical problems 35–6
  other conditions 24–5
  redness 31, 33
  scratching 31, 33
  skin care 46
  symptoms 32–4
azathioprine 74

B
B complex vitamins 120
bacteria 13, 19, 42, 70
balance
  Chinese philosophy 81–2, 86
  diet 101–2
bananas 102, 109
bandages 72–3
bathing 27, 50, 58, 88
beans 102
beds 54–5
beef 109
beta-carotene 102, 120
birthdays 29
bleaches 37, 49
blinds 54–5
blisters 32–3
blood
  tests 110

vessels 16–18, 21
  white cells 74
blow heaters 55
blushing 17
bones 21
bread 102
breast-feeding 116, 118
breathing 97
broccoli 102, 120
brown rice 102
bruising 69
bullying 61
burdock 89

C
cabbage 102
caffeine 103–4, 108
calamine 73
calcium 19, 21, 116
calendula 89
capsules 88
carbohydrates 102
carbon dioxide 13, 20
care, skin 45–52, 70
carpets 54
carrots 102, 120
causes, eczema 26–7
cautions, dietary measures 100
cells
  immune cells 13, 15
  keratinocytes 13–15
  Langerhans 15
  mast 28
  melanocytes 14–15
  Merkel 15
  white blood cells 74
cement 37, 38
central heating 52, 54–5, 58
challenge phase, exclusion diets 112
chamomile 89
cheeses 103–4, 109
chemicals

chlorine 49–50
chromate 38
  household 27, 37, 58
  phyto-chemicals 101
  school issues 63
chi 81, 86
chickweed 89
children
  atopic eczema 25, 30–1, 60
  avoiding irritants 63
  baby milks 116–17
  birthdays 29
  breast-feeding 118
  Chinese herbalism 87
  diet 30, 114–16
  eczema causes 26–7
  exclusion diets 111
  food sensitivities 105, 107–8
  food supplements 113
  growth factors 68
  herbal treatments 84
  hyperactivity 72
  hypnosis 94
  immediate food hypersensitivity 105
  infections 95
  over-protection 30
  school 62–3
  severe atopic eczema 30
  sleep 72–3
  stress 60
  symptoms control 60–3
  topical steroids 69
  treats 116
  triggers 29
  weaning 118–19
  wet wrap dressings 72–3
Chinese herbalism 85–7

Chinese philosophy 81–2, 86
chlorine 49–50
chocolate 104, 109, 119
chromate 38
chronic actinic eczema *see* light-sensitive eczema
cigarette smoke 27, 29–30, 49, 58
citrus fruits 109, 119–20
clams 103, 120
cleaning advice 55
clear film dressings 73
climate changes 58
clothing 51–2
coal-tar 73–5
cocoa 103, 120
codes of practice 97
coffee 103–4, 109
cola-type drinks 103–4
cold sores 42, 62
colds 26
collagen 16, 21
command hypnotherapy 93
complementary treatments 77–98
    acupuncture 81–3
    allergy tests 110
    first appointments 80
    herbal treatments 84–9
    homeopathy 90–3
    hypnosis 93–4
    naturopathy 94–5
    physical therapies 96–7
    reflexology 96
    safety 97–8
    therapists 79–80
    therapy choice 80–1
    usage 78–9
    yoga 96–7

complexity, herb chemistry 88
complications, eczema 41–2
compresses 88, 89
constipation 107
constitutional remedies 90–1
constriction, blood vessels 17
consultations
    acupuncture 82–3
    herbal treatments 88
    homeopathy 92–3
    hypnosis 94
contact dermatitis 36–8
contraceptive pill 58
convector heaters 55
coolness 52
corn 108
corticosteroids *see* steroids
cortisol 56, 67–8
cortisone 19
cosmetics 27, 49
costs, United Kingdom 23–4
cotton 51
courgettes 102
couscous 102
cow's milk 105, 109, 115–19
cracked skin 37
cradle cap 39
cravings 107
creams 47–9
    anti-histamines 71
    herbal treatments 88
    steroids 68
cyclosporine 74

D
daily regimens 49
dairy products 102–3, 109, 115
damp 29

dander 30, 55, 109
dandruff 39
decoctions 85, 88
deep relaxation 93–4
dehumidifiers 29
delayed food hypersensitivity 106–7
demographic issues 23–4
depression 107
dermal papillae 15–16
dermatitis 24
dermis 12, 15–16, 18
detergents 37, 58
dhyana, hatha yoga 97
diagnoses 46
diarrhoea 107, 115
diary-keeping 57–9, 76, 108
diet 8–9
    cautions 100
    children 30, 114–16
    diets 110–14
    eczema prevention 117–18
    healthy skin 103
    herbal consultations 89
    naturopathy 95
    tests 110–14
    treatments 114–17
digestive system 20, 105
digitalis 84
discoid eczema 40
doctors 76, 98
dressings 75
drowsiness 72
    see also tiredness
drugs
    azathioprine 74
    cortisone 19
    cyclosporine 74
    individual treatments 66
    irritants 105

psoralen 75
steroids 67–9, 120
triggers 58, 105
dryness 25, 31, 33, 120
dust 49, 58
dust mites *see* house
dust mites
duvets 54

E
echinacea 89
eczema 23–43
allergic reactions
27–8
atopic eczema 30–6
causes 26–7
complications 41–2
contact dermatitis
36–8
control 45–63
eczema herpeticum
42
herbal treatments 89
homeopathic
remedies 92
prevention 28–30,
117–18
professional
organizations 81
symptoms 25–6,
32–4, 45–63
types 30–41
Eczema in childhood:
the facts (Atherton)
86
eczema craquele *see*
asteatotic eczema
effectiveness,
homeopathy 91
eggs 102–3, 105,
108–9, 115,
118–20
elasticity, skin 16, 69
elder flowers 89
elimination diets *see*
exclusion diets

emollients 46–9, 66
emulsifying ointment
49
environmental factors
27–9
epidermis 12–15
erythema *see* redness
evening primrose oil
113
exclusion diets 95, 107,
110–14
exclusion recipes
121–71
exfoliating scrubs 50
exhaust fumes 27
eyes 32, 34, 105

F
family history 80
fasting 95, 111
fats 103–4
feathers 26, 54
fertilizers 37
fingernails 59
fingerprints 16
fish 102–3, 108–9,
118–20
Fitzgerald, William 96
five elements, Chinese
philosophy 82
flakes, skin 26
floors 54
fluid retention 107
flushes 17, 107
follicles, hair 16
food intolerance *see*
delayed food
hypersensitivity
foods 99–120
action points 107–9
additives 48, 109
atopic eczema 30
causes of eczema 26
diary-keeping 108
irritant contact
dermatitis 37

labels 115
school issues 63
sensitivities 104–7
skin 101–4
supplements 113
tests 110–14
treatments 114–17
triggers 56, 58,
108–9
urticaria 34–5
forecasts, pollen 53
foxgloves 84
free-radicals 102,
120
fruit acids 50
fruits 50, 102–3,
108–9, 119–20
fungi 26, 42
furnishings 54–5

G
game 102
gamma linoleic acid
(GLA) 113
gels 68
genetic factors 24,
26–7
GLA *see* gamma linoleic
acid
glands 16–18, 25,
35–6, 68
gloves 51, 59, 73
glucocorticoids *see*
steroids
goat's milk 116
graphites 92
gravitational eczema
25, 41
Great Ormond Street
Hospital for Sick
Children 86, 111
Group A *Streptococcus*
70
growth factors 35, 68,
116
gut walls 105

H

hair 16, 38, 110
hand protection 51
hatha yoga 96–7
hay fever 25, 27, 35, 53
headaches 107
healing crises 98
healthy eating recipes
173–220
heart 21
heat regulation 16–18,
20, 25
hepatitis 87
herbal pharmacists 87
herbal treatments 84–9
Chinese herbalism
85–7
medical herbalism
87–8
herpes simplex virus 42
herrings 103
histamine 28, 34, 70–2,
103, 105
hives 34
homeopathy 90–3
homeostasis 16
homes 52, 54
hormone replacement
therapy (HRT) 58
hormones
body systems 21
cortisol 67–8
HRT 58
sex 21
stress 56–7
hospitalization 75
house dust mites
genetic factors 26
keratinocytes 14
skin prick tests 109
triggers 14, 29–30,
54–5, 58
vacuuming 55
household chemicals
27, 37, 58
see also chemicals

HPV see human
papillomavirus
HRT see hormone
replacement therapy
human papillomavirus
(HPV) 42
humidity factors 29,
32, 40, 52
hydrocortisone 19, 67,
69
hydrolyzed cow's
milk formula
117–18
hydrotherapy 95
hyperactivity 72
hypnosis 93–4
hypoallergenic
products 48
hypodermis 12–13
hypoglycaemia 107

I

ice-packs 60
ichthammol 75
IgE see
Immunoglobulin E
illnesses 57–8
immediate food
hypersensitivity
105–6, 115
immune system
herbal consultations
89
herbal treatments 85
immune cells 13, 15
omega-6 fatty acids
120
proteins 102
sensitization 28
skin 21
steroids 67
stress 56–7
Immunoglobulin E
antibody test see
radioallergosorbent
test

Immunoglobulin E (IgE)
27–8, 105
immunosuppressive
drugs 73–4
indigestion 107
individual treatments
Chinese herbalism
85–7
complementary
treatments 78
homeopathy 90–1
orthodox treatments
66
infantile atopic eczema
31, 60
infections
children 95
eczema causes 26–7
eczema
complications
41–2
irritants 27
nummular eczema
40
orthodox treatments
65–6
scratching 19
vitamins A/C 120
inflammation
contact dermatitis 38
dermatitis 24, 38
omega-3 fatty acids
120
prostaglandins 104
reflexology 96
skin 32
steroids 67
infusions 88
Ingham, Eunice 96
intestinal eczema 36
irritability 107
irritant contact
dermatitis 37
irritants
see also triggers
alcohol 27

avoidance 49
bathing 27
bleaches 37, 49
cement 37
chemicals 49, 63
chlorine 50
cigarette smoke 27,
   49, 58
cosmetics 27, 49
detergents 37, 58
dust 49, 58
exhaust fumes 27
fertilizers 37
foods 37, 63
household chemicals
   27, 37, 58
infections 27
leaky gut walls 105
medical herbalism 89
metals 51
mineral oils 49
occupational
   dermatitis 24
over-exertion 27
overheating 27,
   63
paint 37
perfumes 49
sand 49, 58
school issues 63
soap 49, 58, 63
soil 37
solvents 49
sports 63
stress 27
swimming 63
synthetic fibres 49,
   51, 58
textiles 27
trauma 27
water 37, 63
wool 49, 51, 58
itchiness
   atopic eczema 31–3
   B complex vitamins
      120

delayed food
   hypersensitivity 107
eczema symptoms
   25, 28
eyes 105
hypnosis 93–4
Immunoglobulin E
   28
itch-scratch cycle 31,
   59–60, 71–2
school issues 62

J
jaundice 87
joint aches 107

K
Kaposi's varicelliform
   eruption see eczema
   herpeticum
keratinization 33–4
keratinocytes 13–15,
   35
keratosis pilaris 31
kidney damage 74
kinesiology 110

L
labels 48, 115
lactose tablets 90
lamb and pears diet
   111
Langerhans cells 15
lanolin 38, 48
lawns 53
leaky gut walls 105
lettuce 102
lichen-simplex 41
lichenification 31–2, 34
light therapy 75
light-sensitive eczema
   40
linseed oil 113
liver function 86–7
lotions 47–9, 68, 71,
   75

lungs 20
lymph nodes 35

M
management
   childhood eczema
      61–2
   eczema symptoms
      45–63
mangoes 112
marigold 89
masked food allergy see
   delayed food
   hypersensitivity
masks 55
massage 95
mast cells 28
mattresses 54
meat 102–3
medical issues
   diagnosis 46
   medical herbalism
      87–8
   MedicAlert bracelets
      36
   medications 58, 66,
      105
meditation 97
melanin 13–15, 18,
   33
melanocytes 14–15
menopause 21, 57–8
menstruation 58
Merkel cells 15
metabolic processes
   18–19
metals 38, 51
milk 105–6, 108–9,
   115–19
mineral oils 49
minerals 20, 49, 113
'miracle' cures 98
mites see house dust
   mites
moisturizers 46–9,
   59–60, 66

molluscum
contagiosum 42
mother tincture,
homeopathy 90
moulds 30, 109
multi-vitamin
supplements 113
muscles 20, 107, 110

N
nail damage 34
National Eczema
Society 115
National Health Service
86
naturopathy 94–5
needle insertion,
acupuncture 83
nerves 16–17, 20, 59
nettle rash 32, 34
nettles 89
neurodermatitis 41
nickel 51
nipples 32
nummular eczema 40
nuts 103, 105, 108–9,
118–20

O
oats 108, 120
occupational dermatitis
24
oil free products 48
oil glands 16–17
oil-in-water emulsions
48
oils
evening primrose
113
sebum 13, 19, 21,
37, 46
vegetable oils 103,
113, 120
ointments
anti-histamines 71
herbal treatments 88

moisturizers 47–9
steroids 68
omega-3 fatty acids
103, 120
omega-6 fatty acids
103, 120
oral steroids 68
organizations, eczema
81, 97, 115
orthodox treatments
65–76
anti-histamines 70–2
antibiotics 70
antiseptics 70
bandages 72–3
Chinese herbalism 86
emollient therapy 66
hospitalization 75
immunosuppressive
drugs 73–4
individual treatments
66
light therapy 75
naturopathy 95
tar preparations
74–5
osteopathy 95
osteoporosis 68
over-exertion 27
over-protection 30,
60–1
overheating 27, 63
oxygen 13, 20–1
oysters 103, 120

P
paint 37
pallid skin 33
Pantajali 96
papaya 112, 120
papillae, dermal 15–16
parental advice 29–30
pasta 102
patch tests 48
peanuts 105, 108–9,
119

peas 102
peppers 102
perfumes 38, 49
petroleum 50, 52, 92
pets 26, 55–6
pharmacists 87
photosensitive eczema
see light-sensitive
eczema
phototherapy see light
therapy
physical examinations
80
physical therapies
96–7
phyto-chemicals 101
picture books 61
pigmentation 33
the pill 58
plantains 102
plants 38, 53, 75
PMS see premenstrual
symptoms
pollens 26, 29–30, 53,
109
pompholyx eczema see
vesicular eczema
pork 109
postures, hatha yoga
97
potatoes 102
poultices 88
poultry 102, 109
pranayama, yoga 97
pregnancy
diary-keeping 57–8
eczema causes 26
eczema prevention
117–18
herbal treatments
84
skin changes 21
triggers 29
premenstrual
symptoms (PMS) 57
preservatives 38

pressure points 96
pressure whitening 33
prevention, eczema
28–30, 117–18
professional
organizations 97, 115
prostaglandins 104
protection, skin 12–13
proteins 102, 105, 116
proving homeopathic
remedies 93
psoralen 75
psoriasis 19, 34–5
psychotherapy 95
pulses 83
pumpkin seeds 103

Q

qualifications,
therapists 79
quercetins 102, 120
questions, doctors 76

R

radioallergosorbent test
(RAST) 106, 110
rare foods diet 111
rashes 31–2, 38, 65,
80, 115
RAST see
radioallergosorbent
test
recipes 121–220
red clover 89
redness
atopic eczema 31, 33
dietary treatments
115
eczema effects 25
immediate food
hypersensitivity
105
Immunoglobulin E 28
psoriasis 35
seborrhoeic eczema
39

reflexology 96
regimens, moisturizing
49
Register of Chinese
Herbal Medicine 87
regulations, treatments
79
relaxation 93
reproductive systems
21, 57–8
research
Chinese herbalism
85–6
genetic factors 27
homeopathy 91
rhinitis 25, 27, 35
rice 102, 106, 119–20
Riley, Joe 96
rubber 38
runny noses 35, 115
rye 108, 120

S

safety issues 67, 84,
97–8
safflower oil 113
salami 103–4
salmon 103, 120
sand 49, 58
sardines 103, 120
saturated fats 103–4
sausages 103–4
scabs 38
scaly skin 25, 33, 39
school issues 62–3
scientific explanations,
homeopathy 91
scratching
atopic eczema 31, 33
dietary treatments
115
infections 19
itch-scratch cycle
59–60, 71–2
seborrhoeic eczema 39,
120

sebum 13, 19, 21, 37,
46
seeds 103, 120
selenium 102
self-adhesive clear film
dressings 73
self-help groups 97
self-management,
children 61
self-treatments 91
sensations 16, 18, 83
sensitivities, foods
99–100, 104–7
sensitization steps 28
sensory receptors
16–18
severe atopic eczema 30
sex hormones 21
shellfish 108–9
'shiners' 34
side effects
anti-histamines 71
immunosuppressive
drugs 74
light therapy 75
medical herbalism 88
steroids 68–9
skin 11–21, 45–52
care 45–52, 70
cracking 37
dermis 15–16
dietary advice 103
eczema
complications
41–2
epidermis 13–15
facts 17
foods 101–4
immune system 21
inflammation 24, 32
nutrients table 120
pallidness 33
pigmentation 33
pregnancy 21
pressure whitening
33

protection 12–13
scaly skin 25, 33, 39
skin prick tests
    109–10
steroids 69
thickening 33
weepiness 32, 48
sleep 72–3
smoking 29
sneezing 105
soap 49, 58, 63
socks 51
softeners, water 50
soil 37
solids, weaning 118–19
solvents 49
sore throats 70
sores 38
soya 108–9, 116–17,
    120
spinach 102, 120
spores 26
sports 63
squash 102
Staphylococcus aureus
    42, 70
stasis eczema 25, 41
steroids 67–9
    omega-6 fatty acids
        120
    oral steroids 68
    topical steroids 68–9
strengths
    homeopathy
        remedies 90
    topical steroids 68–9
Streptococcus, Group A
    70
stress
    atopic eczema 30
    B complex vitamins
        120
    childhood eczema 60
    complementary
        treatments 77–8
    hormones 56–7

hypnosis 93
irritants 27
leaky gut walls 105
physical therapies
    96–7
reflexology 96
triggers 56–7, 97
yoga 97
stretch marks 16, 69
sugary foods 103
sulphur 92
sunflower oil 113, 120
sunlight 15, 18–19,
    40
supplements 58, 113
sweat 16–18, 21, 107
sweet potatoes 112,
    120
swelling 28, 32, 35,
    105
swimming 50, 58, 63
symptoms
    atopic eczema 32–4
    delayed food
        hypersensitivity
        106–7
    eczema 25–6, 32–4
    Immunoglobulin E
        28
    menopause 57
    premenstrual
        symptoms 57
symptoms control
    45–63
    avoiding irritants 49
    children 60–3
    moisturizers 46–9
    skin care 45–52
    triggers 52–8
    water avoidance 50
synthetic fibres 49, 51,
    58

T
tablets 88, 90
tar preparations 73–5

TCM *see* traditional
    Chinese medicine
teas 85, 88, 103–4,
    109, 120
tests
    allergies 109–14
    blood tests 110
    complementary
        treatments 110
    exclusion diets
        110–14
    radioallergosorbent
        test 106, 110
    skin prick tests
        109–10
textiles 27
therapists 79–80
thickened skin 33, 35
thirst 20, 25
tights 51
tinctures 88, 90
tiredness 58, 62, 72
tomatoes 102
topical drugs 19, 68–9
touch 15–16
towelling 50
toxins 96–7
traditional Chinese
    medicine (TCM)
    81, 85
training, therapists 79
trances 93–4
trauma 27
treatments
    complementary
        77–98, 110
    diets 114–17
    orthodox 65–76, 86,
        95
treats 116
triggers
    see also allergens:
        irritants
    breast-feeding 118
    Chinese philosophy
        82

common triggers 58,
108–9
diary-keeping 57–8,
76
drugs 58, 105
eczema prevention
29
elimination 52–6
environmental
factors 27–9
foods 56, 58, 108–9
house dust mites 14,
54–5
identification 52–6
pets 55–6
pollen 53
pregnancy 117–18
stress 56–7, 97
trust 79–80
tummy aches 25, 36
tuna 103, 120
turkey 111

U
UK see United Kingdom
ultraviolet radiation
(UV) 13, 15, 40, 75
United Kingdom (UK)
Chinese herbalism 86
demographic issues
23
eczema costs 23–4
homeopathic
consultations 92
National Eczema
Society 115
United States of
America 111
urban living 29, 32

urinary system 18, 21,
26, 36
urticaria 32, 34–5,
105
UV see ultra violet
radiation

V
vacuuming 55
varicose eczema 25, 41
vega testing 110
vegetable oils 103,
113, 120
vegetables 102–3,
119–20
vesicles see blisters
vesicular eczema 39
vibrational patterns
91
viruses
Coxsackie virus 42
herpes simplex virus
42
human
papillomavirus 42
molluscum
contagiosum 42
visualization 93–4
vitamins
A 102, 120
B complex 120
C 102, 120
D 18–19, 20–1
E 102, 120
skin absorbency 13

W
warts 42
water 37, 50, 63

water-in-oil emulsions
48
weaning 118–19
'wear and tear'
dermatitis 37
weeping skin 32, 48
Western herbalism
87–8
wet wrap dressings 72
wheat 105–6, 108–9,
119–20
wheezing 105
white blood cells 74
white fish 108–9
white willow bark 84
whitened skin 33
whole-person
prescribing 77, 80,
91
wholemeal bread 102
willow bark 84
wind 107
wine 103–4
witch hazel 89
wool 49, 51, 58
wraps 72–3

Y
yams 102, 111
yarrow 89
yeasts 19, 108–9, 120
yellow dock 89
yin and yang 82, 86
yoga 96–7

Z
zinc 103, 113, 120
zone therapy 96

Recipe Index

A

Andalusian chicken
210–11
apple and walnut salad
181
artichokes provençal
145

B

baked herrings with
ginger and honey
sauce 200–1
beans, peas and lentils
chickpea and tomato
rice 154–5
chilled pea soup 122
chilli bean and
pepper soup 123
dhal 194–5
green pea stew with
saffron and mint
190–1
hearty bean soup
178–9
beef, stir-fried with
peppers 220
beetroot risotto
150–1
brown rice with mixed
herbs 152–3

C

caponata 186–7
carrot and caraway
salad 134–5
Catalan pork stew
216
celeriac and apple soup
174–5
chicken
Andalusian chicken
210–11
chicken en cocotte
214–15
paella with rabbit
and chicken 168–9
pesto chicken kebabs
159
stir-fried chicken
with crunchy
vegetables 212–13
chickpea and tomato
rice 154–5
chilled pea soup 122
chilli bean and pepper
soup 124–5
couscous with lamb
218–19
creamy tomato sauce
208
cucumber and
pineapple salad with
guacamole 126–7
curries
madras fish kebabs
206–7

prawn and mango
curry 209
pumpkin curry
138–9

D
dhal 194–5
duck
honey duck breasts
with plum and
mango salsa
156–7
smoked duck and
mango salad 132

F
fiery green salad with
poppadum strips
128–9
fish 196–209
baked herrings with
ginger and honey
sauce 200–1
grilled salmon with
potato cakes and
watercress sauce
198–9
grilled salmon and
scallop salad
136–7
madras fish kebabs
206–7
monkfish in creamy
tomato sauce 208
prawn and mango
curry 209
red mullet with
fennel and rouille
202–3
smoked salmon and
asparagus
fettuccine 196–7
swordfish casserole
204–5
french bean and
apricot salad 130

fresh tomato soup
123

G
ginger and honey
sauce 200–1
green pea stew with
saffron and mint
190–1
grilled dishes
asparagus salad
148–9
pepper salad 133
salmon with potato
cakes and water
cress sauce 198–9
salmon and scallop
salad 136–7
guacamole 126–7

H
ham, turkey and parma
ham kebabs 158
hearty bean soup
178–9
herrings, baked with
ginger and honey
sauce 200–1
honey duck breasts
with plum and
mango salsa 156–7

I
Italian leek and
pumpkin soup 176

J
Jamaican pepperpot
soup 177
jersey royal and celery
salad 131

L
lamb
lamb with couscous
218–19

lamb shanks with
olives, sun-dried
tomatoes and
saffron mash
162–3
lamb and vegetable
hotpot 165
marinated lamb
kebabs 160–1
noisettes of lamb
with savoury
butter 164
lentils see beans, peas
and lentils
liver, stir-fried liver and
spinach with ginger
217

M
madras fish kebabs
206–7
marinated lamb kebabs
160–1
meat 160–71, 216–20
Catalan pork stew
216
lamb with couscous
218–19
lamb shanks with
olives, sun-dried
tomatoes and
saffron mash
162–3
lamb and vegetable
hotpot 165
marinated lamb
kebabs 160–1
noisettes of lamb
with savoury
butter 164
paella with rabbit
and chicken 168–9
rabbit with rosemary
and mustard
170–1
spicy pork rolls with

minted yogurt 166–7

stir-fried beef with peppers 220

stir-fried liver and spinach with ginger 217

monkfish in creamy tomato sauce 208

mullet, red mullet with fennel and rouille 202–3

N

navarin of spring vegetables 142–3

noisettes of lamb with savoury butter 164

noodles
noodles with chinese vegetables 192–3
rice noodle soup 180

P

pasta
provençal pasta salad 182
smoked salmon and asparagus fettuccine 196–7
tagliatelle sicilienne 183

peas *see* beans, peas and lentils

pesto chicken kebabs 159

plum and mango salsa 156–7

pork
Catalan stew 216
spicy pork rolls with minted yogurt 166–7

potatoes
grilled salmon with potato cakes and

watercress sauce 198–9

jersey royal and celery salad 131

potato cakes 198–9

scalloped potatoes 188–9

poultry 156–9, 168–9, 210–15
Andalusian chicken 210–11
chicken en cocotte 214–15
honey duck breasts with plum and mango salsa 156–7
paella with rabbit and chicken 168–9
pesto chicken kebabs 159
stir-fried chicken with crunchy vegetables 212–13
turkey and parma ham kebabs 158

prawn and mango curry 209

provençal pasta salad 182

pumpkin curry 138–9

R

rabbit
paella with rabbit and chicken 168–9
rabbit with rosemary and mustard 170

ratatouille niçoise 146–7

red mullet with fennel and rouille 202–3

rice
beetroot risotto 150–1

brown rice with mixed herbs 152–3

chickpea and tomato rice 154–5

paella with rabbit and chicken 168–9

rice noodle soup 180

yellow rice with mushrooms 184

roille 202–3

root vegetable bake 185

S

salads 126–37, 181–2
apple and walnut salad 181
carrot and caraway salad 134–5
cucumber and pineapple salad with guacamole 126–7
fiery green salad with poppadum strips 128
french bean and apricot salad 130
grilled asparagus salad 148–9
grilled pepper salad 133
grilled salmon and scallop salad 136–7
jersey royal and celery salad 131
provençal pasta salad 182
smoked duck and mango salad 132

salmon
grilled salmon with potato cakes and watercress sauce 198–9

grilled salmon and scallop salad 136–7
smoked salmon and asparagus fettuccine 196–7
sauces
creamy tomato sauce 208
ginger and honey sauce 200–1
roille 202–3
watercress sauce 198–9
savoury butter 164
scalloped potatoes 188–9
scallops, grilled salmon and scallop salad 136–7
smoked dishes
duck and mango salad 132
salmon and asparagus fettuccine 196–7
soups 122–5, 174–80
celeriac and apple soup 174–5
chilled pea soup 122
chilli bean and pepper soup 124–5
fresh tomato soup 123
hearty bean soup 178–9
Italian leek and pumpkin soup 176
Jamaican pepperpot soup 177
rice noodle soup 180
spicy pork rolls with minted yogurt 166–7
spicy roasted vegetables 140–1

stir-fried dishes
beef with peppers 220
chicken with crunchy vegetables 212–13
liver and spinach with ginger 217
vegetables 144
swordfish casserole 204

T
tagliatelle sicilienne 183
tomatoes
chickpea and tomato rice 154–5
fresh tomato soup 123
lamb shanks with olives, sun-dried tomatoes and saffron mash 162–3
monkfish in creamy tomato sauce 208
turkey and parma ham kebabs 158

V
vegetables 138–55, 183–95
artichokes provençal 145
beetroot risotto 150–1
brown rice with mixed herbs 152–3
caponata 186–7
carrot and caraway salad 134–5
chickpea and tomato rice 154–5
chilled pea soup 122
chilli bean and pepper soup 124

dhal 194–5
fresh tomato soup 123
green pea stew with saffron and mint 190–1
grilled asparagus salad 148–9
hearty bean soup 178–9
Italian leek and pumpkin soup 176
Jamaican pepperpot soup 177
jersey royal and celery salad 131
navarin of spring vegetables 142–3
noodles with chinese vegetables 192–3
potato cakes 198–9
pumpkin curry 138–9
ratatouille niçoise 146–7
root vegetable bake 185
scalloped potatoes 188–9
spicy roasted vegetables 140–1
stir-fried vegetables 144
tagliatelle sicilienne 183
watercress sauce 198–9
yellow rice with mushrooms 184

W
watercress sauce 198–9

Y
yellow rice with mushrooms 184